Scottish Home and Health Departme

Scottish Health Authorities Priorities for the Eighties

A Report by the Scottish Health Service Planning Council

ISBN 0 11 491689 6

Foreword by the Secretary of State for Scotland

I am grateful to the Scottish Health Service Planning Council for preparing such a thorough and comprehensive report on the priorities for the health services in Scotland in the 1980s.

I agree with the Council's assessment of priorities as summarised in paragraphs VI.20 and VI.21 of the Report. This involves giving high priority to prevention and to the development of services for patients requiring long term care. I am asking health boards and the Common Services Agency to take account and, where appropriate in the light of their local situation, to make allocations of resources according to the assessment of relative priorities set out in this Report.

The Council have put prevention at the top of their list of priorities. Much of the damage to the health of the Scottish people is self-inflicted by smoking and excessive drinking. It is very important to do all we can by health education and other means to promote healthy living and to reduce the number of people who have avoidable recourse to health care.

The Council have also emphasised the importance of services for the elderly and have made special mention of the needs of the elderly with mental disability. Everyone knows about the increasing proportion of the very elderly in our population; and it is essential that in our plans for health services we do all we can to provide suitable care for this group of patients.

It has to be understood, of course, that the Council's recommendations relate to the broad pattern of need over Scotland as a whole. Granted the different pattern of services in different parts of the country and the extent to which they already provide for the needs of various groups of patients, the Council's recommendations will have to be interpreted in the light of local requirements.

The availability of finance will govern, as the Council themselves recognise, the extent to which services can be developed. Whatever the level of resources available in the years ahead, the Council's Report forms a valuable basis for consideration of the way in which the available money should be spent; and I hope that it will be read carefully by all concerned with health services in Scotland.

George Younger.

New St. Andrew's House
EDINBURGH.
December, 1980.

NOTE BY PROFESSOR E. M. McGIRR, CBE, CHAIRMAN, SCOTTISH HEALTH SERVICE PLANNING COUNCIL

A report on health priorities in Scotland for the 1980s was prepared for the Council by its Working Party on Health Priorities. After being adjusted in a number of relatively minor ways to take account both of the Council's views and of the views of the National Consultative Committees, it was adopted by the Council. The report which is now printed is the report as sent by the Council to the Secretary of State in May of this year.

The Council is grateful for the work done by the Working Party under its Chairman, Mr J. G. Wallace, OBE. A copy of the preface prepared by Mr Wallace for the Council, covering the Working Party's original report, and a list of members of the Working Party appear at Appendices 3 and 4.

Contents

I The Need for Health Care

Introduction

I.1 Ideally the provision of health services should be related to the need for health care, which is in turn largely determined by disease and disability in the population and the size and structure of the population itself. Population structure is important both because mortality and morbidity in the population depend on the respective sizes of different age/sex groups which have different mortality/morbidity rates, and because some health services are specific to particular age groups, eg paediatric services. However, additional demands can be created by the discovery and development of treatments for conditions which were previously irremediable, eg the introduction of hip joint replacement in orthopaedic surgery; or needs can be reduced by preventive measures. The population's health will be affected by many factors outwith the NHS (eg housing standards) and the pressure on the NHS will be affected by the availability of alternative provision (eg residential homes).

(A) MORBIDITY

I.2 In the absence of satisfactory means of measuring the health of the population the best that can be done is to take the indicators of ill health, namely, morbidity and mortality, and consider them over time. Morbidity is the preferable measure, but the only morbidity data currently available which are not based upon contacts with the health or other services come from the General Household Survey. This Survey shows that the rates for acute and chronic illness are higher for women than men, and also vary with age. Rates for acute illness are relatively high for the under fives and then fall for older children before rising steadily with age to the over 75s. The rates for chronic illness (which is more likely to create a need for long-term care) also rise with age but more steeply, and the difference between old and young is much more marked than for acute illness. Rates for acute illness may be rising,

1

but the evidence is inconclusive, and no comparisons over time are possible for chronic illness. *Better morbidity data would improve health planning and monitoring and consideration should be given to possible means of improving the Scottish data in this respect.*

(B) MORTALITY

I.3 In the absence of wholly satisfactory data on morbidity, an alternative approach is to use available data on mortality as a proxy, bearing in mind that there are substantial limitations on their value in this context. During this century Scottish mortality rates have improved enormously, though the improvement has been much more marked for infants and younger adults than for the elderly. The higher life expectancy of females means that more elderly women are likely to be widowed and living alone, and thus are more likely to require long-term care.

I.4 Despite the considerable improvement in the Scottish mortality rates, they remain high compared with other developed countries. The Scottish figures are worse than those for England and Wales, and if comparisons are drawn with developed countries in the Organisation for Economic Co-operation and Development, Scotland is the fourth worst of 24 countries[1] for male life expectancy and second worst for female life expectancy, but around the average for infant mortality. International comparisons must be treated with caution, but there can be no doubt that Scotland's experience is unsatisfactory. Many deaths, moreover, are premature, resulting as they do from bad habits such as abuse of alcohol and smoking; therefore in Chapter V the role of health education in modifying such behaviour is considered.

I.5 There has been little improvement in mortality difference between social classes, with Social Classes IV and V continuing to fare much worse than Classes I and II. These differences may be difficult to eradicate, since they may reflect not only differences in behaviour and lifestyle but also the tendency of people in poor health to slide down the social class scale. Implementation of the recommendations on multiple deprivation and prevention in Chapters IV and V, and on ante-natal care in relation to perinatal mortality in Chapter II, should help to close the gap.

---

[1]For purposes of this comparison Turkey and Yugoslavia were excluded; England and Wales were included.

I.6 There are differences in standardised mortality ratios (SMR) between health boards, with the worst rates in 1977 being found in the four health boards covering Strathclyde Region. Persistent differences between boards may be due, at least in part, to differences in social class composition and the proportion of a board's population which is multiply deprived. SMRs have been adopted by the SHARE Working Party as measuring differing needs for health care. On this assumption, these differing needs are taken into account in the distribution of financial revenue resources to health boards.

(C) POPULATION

I.7 The Scottish home population has fluctuated only slightly around the present figure of 5.2 million since 1961 and no significant change is expected in the years up to 1991. At national level therefore changes in the age/sex structure of the population will be much more important from a NHS viewpoint than changes in its size. Both the size and the structure of a population are determined by three factors: present or past fertility, migration and mortality. Mortality is reasonably predictable, and at national level variations in net migration currently have a relatively small effect. The main uncertainty about the future Scottish population stems from the birth rate, which will not affect the projections for age groups over 15 (see Table I.1A). Past population changes over the period 1966–77 are also shown in Table I.1A and the corresponding percentages appear in Table I.1B.

Table I.1A Scottish Home Population 1966–1991 by Age Groups

Age Group	1966	1971	1977	1981	1986	1991
0–4 years	482.7	443.4	337.9	308.8	381.4	427.9
5–15 years	940.0	1,001.4	975.1	874.3	738.0	743.2
16–44 years	1,948.9	1,927.2	2,014.8	2,109.5	2,201.9	2,210.3
45–64 years	1,233.5	1,204.2	1,162.6	1,129.8	1,108.0	1,091.3
65–74 years	385.8	424.4	457.7	454.1	428.7	426.1
75–84 years	168.3	181.8	206.0	227.0	244.4	244.6
85+ years	31.2	35.0	41.7	45.5	53.2	61.4
Total Population	5,190.8	5,217.4	5,195.6	5,149.1	5,155.7	5,204.5

Source: Registrar General Scotland–Projected Home Population–1977 Based; and unpublished figures.

Table I.1B Scottish Home Population 1966–1991–Age Groups as % of Whole

Age Group	1966	1971	1977	1981	1986	1991
0–4 years	9.3	8.5	6.5	6.0	7.4	8.2
5–15 years	18.1	19.2	18.8	17.0	14.3	14.3
16–44 years	·37.5	36.9	38.8	41.0	42.7	42.5
45–64 years	23.8	23.1	22.4	21.5	21.5	21.0
65–74 years	7.4	8.1	8.8	8.8	8.3	8.2
75–84 years	3.2	3.5	4.0	4.4	4.7	4.7
85+ years	0.6	0.7	0.8	0.9	1.0	1.2
Total Population	100.0	100.0	100.0	100.0	100.0	100.0

Source: Table I.1A.

NB Due to 'rounding' figures do not always add up to 100%.

I.8 The most important population change is the rise in the number of elderly, ie persons aged 65 years and over. With increasing age greater demands are made upon the acute services and the workload of these services is directly affected by the size of the population aged 65 and over. However the need for long-term care does not reach significant proportions until the age of 75. The demand for long-term care is therefore closely related to the number of persons aged 75 and over and is even more sensitive to the number aged 85 and over. Between 1966 and 1977, all the elderly age groups grew in size and the total elderly population grew by about one-fifth from 585,000 to 705,000. However, between 1977 and 1991 the age group 65–74 is expected to decline by 6.9 per cent, while the numbers aged 75–84 will have increased by 18.7 per cent and those aged 85 and over by no less than 47.2 per cent. This last increase should be kept in perspective as the total number aged over 85 in 1991 will still be only 61,000. This change in the age structure of the elderly towards the oldest age group will increase the demand for long term care, especially for geriatric and psychogeriatric hospital places. It will also increase the demand for acute health care, because the additional demand from those aged 75 and over should outweigh any decline in demand from the slightly smaller numbers in the age group 65–74.

I.9 Births fell from a peak of over 104,000 in 1964 to just over 62,000 in 1977. The effect of this fall took some time to work its way through the child population, and while Table I.1A shows the pre-school population declining since 1966, the 5–15 year old group did not decrease until recent years. Births have been rising since the last quarter of 1976, but according to the Registrar General for Scotland's 1977-based projection,[1] the pre-school population

[1]Registrar General for Scotland: Weekly Return July 1978.

4

will continue to decline until 1981, and the 5–15 age group until 1986, before they rise again; and the total 1991 child population will still be 11 per cent below the 1977 level. For some boards, net migration, which affects the size as well as the structure of a population, will be as important a factor as fertility. For example, Greater Glasgow is expected to lose one-fifth of its population by 1991.

I.10 While only one (central) projection was produced in 1977, the Registrar General for Scotland produced three projections in 1976 – high, central and low variants – to illustrate the effect of differing fertility and birth rate assumptions. The projected live births year by year under these variants and under the 1977 projection are set out in Table I.2, and the implications for the child population are illustrated in Figures I.1A and I.1B. The variations between the births projections are small at first but then show a marked difference. A large divergence between the pre-school projections does not occur until 1981 and not until 1986 for older children. It will be seen that the rise in births has occurred a year earlier than expected in the 1976-based high and central variants, and three years earlier than in the 1976-based low variant. According to the Registrar General for Scotland's figures, three-quarters of the increase between 1977 and 1978 was due to an increase in fertility, and one-quarter to the rising number of women of child-bearing age, and the 1978 fertility levels were above those assumed in the 1976-based central and low variants. On the other hand the total percentage increase in the number of births between 1977 and 1978 was only 3.1 per cent – well within the range of year-to-year fluctuations. It is too soon therefore to say which projection is the most reliable. It should be noted that changes in fertility rates are an important factor and consequently the fertility rate must be kept under close review.

Implications for planning

I.11 The main message which emerges from this study of population is the need for the NHS to be able to adapt to change. While changes in the elderly population are relatively slow and predictable for years ahead, births changes are less predictable and have a more immediate effect so that demands for maternity and child health services fluctuate accordingly. One way of dealing with change is to take resources away from a declining client group and give them to an expanding client group, but this may be difficult, time-consuming and expensive to do, particularly for specialist staff. Moreover, this strategy may be effective only where changes are relatively slow and predictable. The alternative is to plan services in a flexible way so they can deal with a reasonable variety of outcomes.

Table 1.2 Projected Live Births 1976/77 to 1990/1991 in Scotland (thousands)

Year—mid year to mid year		1976/ 77	1977/ 78	1978/ 79	1979/ 80	1980/ 81	1981/ 82	1982/ 83	1983/ 84	1984/ 85	1985/ 86	1986/ 87	1987/ 88	1988/ 89	1989/ 90	1990/ 91
Projection																
1976 Base	High Variant	62.5	62.1*	64.3	70.2	77.9	85.0	89.5	92.8	95.2	96.9	97.9	98.3	98.4†	98.2	97.5
	Central Projection	62.5	61.5*	61.7	63.2	66.4	70.1	74.6	80.3	84.9	87.7	89.2	89.6	89.7†	89.5	88.9
	Low Variant	62.5	61.0	60.2	60.2*	60.6	61.8	63.8	66.2	69.8	73.7	75.9	76.6	76.8†	76.6	76.1
1977 Base	Central Projection	—	62.7*	63.3	64.0	66.3	69.4	73.7	79.3	83.8	86.5	87.9	88.2	88.3†	88.0	87.5
Actual Figures		62.1*†	63.1													

Sources: Working Party on Health Priorities (WPHP) Paper PC1/5/78/15 (unpublished) and R.G. Scotland.

*Low Turning Point.
†High Turning Point.

6

I.12 If the same total amount of resources in real terms continues to be used in a service whose client group is declining, there will be an increase in the resources used per head giving, in effect, increased priority to this client group. This higher priority may not accord with the overall list of priorities adopted for the NHS. Accordingly, consideration should always be given to applying resources which are surplus to requirement to the support of other services with a higher priority.

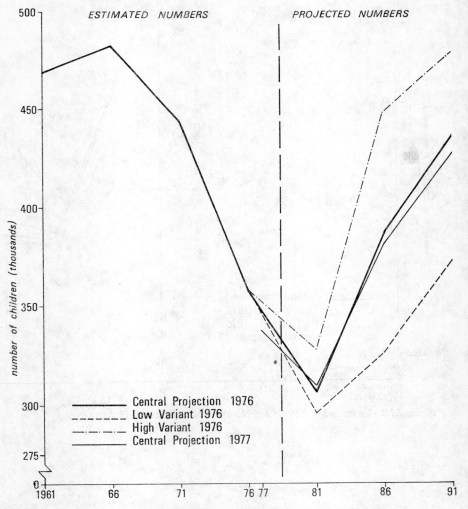

Figure I.1A Estimated and Projected Numbers of Children (0–4 Age Group)

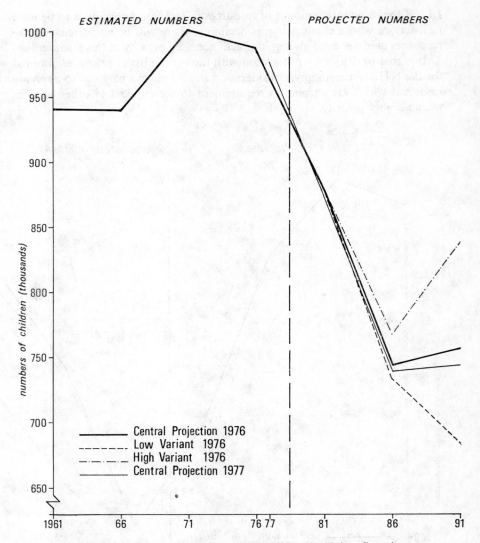

Central Projection 1976
Low Variant   1976
High Variant   1976
Central Projection 1977

Figure I.1B   Estimated and Projected Numbers of Children (5–15 Age Group)

II Provision of Health Care

(A) PRIMARY HEALTH CARE

(i) General medical services

II.1 General medical practitioners provide the point of first contact for patients and they control, to a large extent, the use made of other community services and the hospital service. They are also responsible, through their prescribing, for a large proportion of the national expenditure on pharmaceuticals.

II.2 Since the introduction of the 'Charter for General Practitioners', there has been a steady increase in the numbers of principals in general practice with a consequential fall in the average list size (ie the average number of patients on a principal's list). There were 2,883 principals in practice in 1978 and the average list size was 1,902, compared with 2,572 principals with an average list of 2,068 in 1968. These averages, however, conceal wide variations in actual list sizes, from very small lists in rural areas to very large lists in areas which are unattractive to doctors, eg because of a high percentage of multiply deprived households. Moreover, list size alone does not give an accurate indication of workload; outside commitments, scattered rural lists, or a high proportion of elderly patients on the list are examples of other pertinent factors which have to be considered. Nevertheless, there is no available evidence to suggest that the total number of doctors in general practice is inadequate and it is unlikely that many more will be required in the 1980s. For example, an estimate[1] of the effect of population changes on the number of general practitioner consultations suggests that between 1975 and 1986 they are likely to increase by only 3 per cent.

II.3 *We welcome the commitment to preventive medicine expressed by the National Medical Consultative Committee's Specialty Subcommittee for*

---

[1]Based upon General Household Survey estimates of general practitioner consultation rates and population projections by age and sex.

General Practice. General practitioners are ideally placed with their colleagues in the primary care team to influence patient behaviour and to introduce screening services, such as the developmental screening of children. We hope that preventive medicine will find an increasingly important place in training for general practice and that this aspect of training will include a general practitioner's responsibility for the health education of patients and their families. It is possible that a change in emphasis from treatment to prevention will require an examination of the present contract for general practitioners but that is a matter for the medical profession and the health departments.

II.4 We are pleased to note that the organisation of general practitioners into groups working from health centres or group practice premises has been increasing steadily over the years. In 1965, 41 per cent of general practitioners worked in groups of three or more whereas in 1977 the proportion had risen to 67 per cent. The number of health centres has also grown rapidly and by June 1979 there were 114 in operation, 21 under construction, and 67 at various stages of planning. The formation of primary care teams by the attachment of health visitors and district nurses to general practices is a desirable development, which has still to be fully exploited. The significance of the work of related agencies, particularly social work, is recognised but it is disappointing that only 38 out of 85 health centres covered in a 1976 survey were provided with social work services, and that in only 18 health centres were social workers attached to the primary care teams. It is to be hoped that an expansion of this service will follow the recently introduced policy of making available accommodation in health centres free of charge for social workers providing direct services to the health centre population. *The concept of the primary care team (which includes social work involvement) and the trend towards practitioners working in groups from shared premises should continue to be actively supported.*

(ii) Primary dental care (including dental manpower)

II.5 The extent of the unsatisfactory state of dental health in Scotland was revealed by a survey of Adult Dental Health in 1972, which found that not only was there a higher proportion of Scottish adults without natural teeth than in England and Wales but that the prognosis for people in the 16–34 age group retaining their teeth was poor. Primary responsibility for this is attributable to inadequate daily dental hygiene and, in certain groups, to an abuse of sugar.

II.6 Primary dental care is provided by the General Dental Services, and also by the Community Dental Service who treat the priority classes (children and expectant mothers). The number of treatments carried out by the General Dental Services increased by 40 per cent from 1.69 million to 2.42 million between 1965 and 1977, with a marked increase in conservation work, a doubling of diagnostic X-ray examinations and an increase of 57 per cent in orthodontic treatments. Inspections and treatments provided by the Community Dental Service increased by 12 per cent and 30 per cent respectively over the period 1967 to 1977, again with a shift from extraction to conservation treatments. Although 99 per cent of the Community Dental Service workload relates to children, the majority of children are treated by the General Dental Services.

II.7 The greatest single measure which could be taken to improve dental health and to reduce the demand for dental treatment would be fluoridation of water supplies. Implementation of this measure would reduce the dental caries which children take into adult life by around 50 per cent. It is disappointing therefore that there has not been a greater response by water authorities, whose agreement is required for fluoridation of water supplies, to the unanimous view of health boards that this measure is necessary. We note that the Royal Commission on the NHS has recommended that the Government should introduce legislation *to require water authorities to fluoridate water supplies at the request of health authorities (paragraph 9.60). We strongly support this proposal.* Alternatives to water fluoridation, brushing teeth with fluoride solution or the taking of fluoride tablets, are unlikely to be as effective, because of difficulties in ensuring compliance with such regimes, particularly in the group of children most at risk. *Dental health education programmes aimed at particular groups in the population, ie school children and mothers with young children, may be helpful, but they require evaluation.* In any event, we believe that they will prove to be much less effective than fluoridation.

II.8 Although the provision of dental care has been increasing, it still falls short of the desirable level. Any further increase in provision is dependent on increasing the number of dentists working outside hospital. The total number of dentists has been increasing in recent years, but only at around 1 per cent per annum and the 1977 total of 1,827 on the dental register (including hospital and administrative staff) compares unfavourably with the 2,080 needed to meet the target ratio of 1 to 2,500 population set by the McNair Committee in 1956. Although the amount of private practice by registered dental practitioners is at present believed to be relatively small – we are unable to quantify it precisely – it is understood to be growing and could reduce the availability of primary dental care services within the NHS.

II.9 Dental school intakes are determined on a UK basis, and the scope for improving the situation in Scotland is limited. From 1980 onwards, Scotland may benefit from the increase in intake of students into the Scottish dental schools since 1976 (though not all graduates from these schools will remain in Scotland), but it will still be some years before the McNair target is met. A committee of enquiry set up by the Nuffield Foundation is looking into dental education for the future, including the supply and demand in the various categories of dental manpower and the respective roles of dentists and of dental ancillary staff. There is scope for making greater use of dental hygienists and dental therapists, thus enabling the dentists to concentrate on activities requiring a high level of knowledge and skill, to reduce the effect of the present shortfall. The numbers of such ancillary staff, which are small at present, are increasing only slowly. *Consideration should therefore be given to how their numbers could be expanded more rapidly.*

II.10 The supply of dental technician services is a problem both in terms of obtaining and training manpower: the use of commercial laboratory services is a costly alternative. Consideration might be given by health boards to the development of dental laboratories to provide a service to the Community Dental Service and Dental Hospitals.

II.11 The distribution of dentists working outside hospitals is uneven. The ratio of community dentists and general dental practitioners to population by health board varied in 1977 from 1: 2,765 to 1: 4,161. *Steps should be taken to rectify the uneven availability of dental services.* One step which might help to attract general dental practitioners to areas at present under-provided would be to offer payment on a 'salary plus bonus' basis.

(iii) **General ophthalmic services**

II.12 Three groups of independent contractors provide general ophthalmic services: ophthalmic medical practitioners who carry out sight tests and prescribe only; dispensing opticians who dispense prescriptions only; and ophthalmic opticians (by far the largest group) who test, prescribe and dispense.

II.13 There is a paucity of information about the need for spectacles in the population. Demand, on the other hand, can be measured by the number of sight tests carried out. Although in a few individual years the number of these tests has declined, such falls have occurred less frequently than decreases in the number of prescriptions for spectacles dispensed, which appear to be particularly sensitive to alterations in charges. In addition, many spectacles are supplied privately, either in whole or in part; and the balance between NHS and privately supplied spectacles varies from year to year. Sight tests have increased rapidly in the 1970s, and a projection of this trend into the 1980s suggests that 820,000 tests would be carried out in 1986 compared with 714,000 in 1976.

II.14 Although the number of ophthalmic opticians, who are the normal point of contact between the public and the general ophthalmic services, has declined by 22 per cent from 612 in 1968 to 477 in 1977, there is no evidence to suggest that the general needs of the population are not being met at present. However, specific groups do appear to have problems, namely, the housebound as well as the elderly and the handicapped whether living at home, in local authority residential homes or in long-stay hospitals. These groups, particularly the elderly, can be severely affected by lack of suitable spectacles, and the National Optical Consultative Committee has recently expressed the view that *a domiciliary service is a necessary part of ocular care for the elderly, the handicapped and housebound people.* At present, while domiciliary visits can be arranged by the hospital eye service, there are no formally recognised arrangements for such visits by the general ophthalmic service. However we have been informed that discussions are currently taking place between the health departments and the optical profession concerning the early introduction of a pilot scheme of domiciliary visits for housebound patients. We hope that these will be successful, since *services to the housebound, the elderly and the handicapped, both in the community and in long-stay accommodation, need to be improved.* In advocating such measures we do not wish to imply that current provision for the young and healthy should be diminished.

(iv) General practice pharmaceutical services

II.15 Ninety-seven per cent of medicines prescribed by general medical and dental practitioners are dispensed by general practice pharmacists, who are independent contractors. The remaining 3 per cent are supplied by dispensing doctors who are mostly located in rural areas.

II.16 The number of pharmacies fell from 1,500 in 1965 to 1,136 in 1978, though this fall has been confined to the smaller pharmacies dispensing annually fewer than 20,000 prescriptions. Pharmacies depend on non-NHS business, for example, sale of toiletries, for a large proportion of their income but this proportion has fallen from 60 per cent to 40 per cent over the decade to 1977. This is due to the commercial pressure exercised by other agencies such as supermarkets, and those least able to withstand this pressure have been the smaller pharmacies.

II.17 A recent report on general practice pharmacy[1] presented to us included the suggestion that certain areas adequately supplied by pharmacies should be classified as closed, to induce pharmacies to open in less financially attractive areas. However, particularly in view of the need to attract non-NHS sales, it seems unlikely that 'closure' alone would make such areas attractive to pharmacists. The report recognised this by suggesting financial payments to pharmacies in isolated or financially unattractive areas. However there is no evidence at present to suggest that there is any general scarcity of pharmacies which affects the number of prescriptions dispensed and hence a need for extra financial inducements to be made generally available. Nevertheless, there may be local problems about access to pharmaceutical services which require to be identified and possibly remedied by payments under the 'essential pharmacies allowance'.[2] In order to ensure that such problems are dealt with, *health boards should continue to monitor the availability and distribution of general practice pharmaceutical services at local level.*

II.18 The numbers of prescriptions, the quantity of drugs issued per prescription, and the ingredients of these drugs is almost exclusively in the control of general medical practitioners. From 1965 to 1977, the number of prescriptions dispensed has increased by 31 per cent from 26 million to 34 million. There was also a considerable increase during the same period in the quantity per prescription and, taking this into account, the true increase is nearer 60 per cent. These increases have ocurred despite efforts at economy by the professions and the health departments. In 1977 the cost of these drugs was £55 million. If the trends in the 1965–77 period (not adjusted for increases in quantity) were to be maintained the projected number of prescriptions dispensed in 1986 would lie between 42 million and 44 million. Further strenuous efforts must be made to economise in this field, subject to maintaining adequate standards of patient care.

II.19 We note with approval that steps have already been taken (a) to make general medical practitioners more aware of prescribing, (b) to induce the general public to accept that consultations may not result in prescriptions

---

[1] Report of Working Party on General Practice Pharmacy. Distributed to NHS bodies June 1980.

[2] This allowance is paid from the global sum for general practice pharmaceutical services to assist a pharmacy which is considered necessary but would not otherwise have a large enough income to enable it to be maintained.

and (c) to produce an improved version of the British National Formulary which provides alternative information on drugs to that provided by pharmaceutical firms. However, more requires to be done and we note that the Royal Commission on the NHS has recommended that general practitioners should be required to prescribe by the generic name of the medicine, not by brand name (paragraph 7.44 of the Royal Commission report). This would allow pharmacists to dispense the cheapest version of the drug available. There might be value in regular discussion between general practitioners and pharmacists to achieve more rational prescribing. The Royal Commission has also suggested that a limited list of essential and effective drugs be prepared, excluding ineffective and unnecessarily expensive drugs (paragraph 7.43). The implementation of a limited list system and/or the use of generic prescribing requires more study: but we were pleased to note that the General Practice Subcommittee of the National Medical Consultative Committee supports the preparation of a limited list of essential and effective drugs, though this should be agreed by hospital doctors and GPs in concert rather than being imposed by health boards. *In the meantime, all possible measures should be taken to ensure maximum economy in the drug bill.*

(v) Community nursing services

II.20 Community nursing staff provide district nursing, health visiting, midwifery and school nursing services; in remote areas these services are provided by combined duty nurses.

II.21 The need for community nursing services cannot be measured accurately, though population numbers and structure are a basis for assessing staffing levels. Recommended target ratios on this basis are available for health visitors and district nurses (see paragraph III.16 below) but not for other categories of community nursing staff. Over the past decade there has been a continuing increase in community nursing staff, although in some areas staffing levels still fall below the recommended minimum ratios. In 1977 there was a total of 3,932 field work staff (whole-time equivalent), compared with 2,738 (whole-time equivalent) in 1967.

II.22 Figures on workloads are available in district nursing, health visiting and midwifery, though the workload of combined duty nurses cannot be separately identified. In the period 1967–1977, the district nursing workload increased by around a quarter in terms of cases and by over 40 per cent in terms of visits. During the same period the health visitors' workload (as measured in terms of cases and visits) fell slightly but the nature of their work also changed, due to an increase in the number of attachments to general practice and the development of health centres. The drop in the workload was due to a decrease in the number of expectant mothers and pre-school children, which was only partly offset by an increase in their work with the elderly. The proportion of the total caseload accounted for by the elderly rose from 5 per cent to 17 per cent between 1967 and 1977, and the proportion of total visits made to the elderly from 7 per cent to 20 per cent.

II.23 The work of community-based midwives has changed, due to the fall in the birth rate and to the fact that more than 99 per cent of births now take place in hospital. The major part of their workload now centres on the ante- and post-natal care of mothers, parentcraft teaching and family planning.

II.24 Community nurses have adapted both to changes in the organisation of health care services, and to changes in the community's needs. Their work will continue to be affected by changes in the population structure, particularly the increase in the over 75 age group, and *community nursing services will have to be expanded further to meet the needs of the over 75s.* The community nursing services will also play a key part in the implementation of many of the objectives for the future development of the health service proposed elsewhere in this report. Examples of these are:

(1) *a shift from hospital to community care;*

(2) *more emphasis on preventive measures including health education, and on improving health services for the multiply deprived households;* and

(3) *pilot studies to evaluate the Child Health Programme Planning Group's proposals for improved and regular health surveillance of all children, and the introduction of comprehensive developmental screening programmes for the pre-school child.*

(B) ACUTE HOSPITAL SERVICES

II.25 The acute hospital services provide specialist in-patient and out-patient care for all acute physical illness. Of all the components of the health service, they are the most manpower intensive and involve the greatest use of support services. In 1976/77 the acute hospital services alone accounted for 52 per cent of hospital revenue expenditure. While this may seem substantial in comparison with the resources used for facilities specific to the needs of particular client groups, it must be remembered that each group makes a demand to a greater or lesser extent on the acute services. For example, 27.6 per cent of all discharges from and deaths in acute hospital beds in 1977 and 43.6 per cent of all bed days spent in them were attributable to those over the age of 65.

II.26 Table II.1 summarises the changes which have occurred in the use of in-patient services in the major specialties over the past 10 years. While this gives an indication of need, it must be borne in mind that actual need could only be measured by the prevalence and severity of disease in the population. Complete data of this sort are not available. In addition, caution must be applied in the interpretation of the indices employed. For instance, the number of discharges, which may be taken to indicate the use of services, measures only numbers of patients and not the volume of services supplied; it is also affected by extraneous factors such as the availability of convalescent and other beds to which patients can be transferred and of facilities for patient care in the community. The size of waiting lists depends on a variety of factors and the absolute numbers are of little statistical value, though changes in numbers are to some extent indicative. We did not examine waiting times for an out-patient appointment, but we note that the Royal Commission on the NHS has suggested that waiting times might be just as, or more, significant (paragraph 10.7). Annual throughput per bed, comprising as it does the two elements of length of stay and turnover interval, may provide a useful comparative index of performance between units working in the same specialty.

II.27 It can be seen from Table II.1 that for all in-patients the number of discharges has risen by 2.6 per cent over the 10 year period but this conceals a number of fluctuations. Waiting lists have increased by 3.3 per cent. Despite a fall in the total numbers of available beds by 17 per cent, there has been an increase in throughput of 24 per cent. This is largely due to improved clinical practices which have resulted in a fall in duration of stay in hospital from 13.7 days to 10.6 days (22.6 per cent). The turnover interval has fallen by 7.1 per cent from 4.2 to 3.9 days.

II.28 The outstanding feature of these statistics is the substantial increase in the number on the waiting list for orthopaedics and it is pertinent to note that the National Medical Consultative Committee, in their report on the Acute Hospital Services, have drawn particular attention to this specialty and the need for increased services. In general, there has been a slight increase in the use of in-patient facilities in all specialties except ENT and paediatric surgery.

II.29 There has been relatively little change in the number of out-patient attendances per 1,000 population between 1970 and 1977 for the specialist

Table II.1 Acute Services–In-patient 1967–1977

	No. of Patients Discharged	Percentage Bed Occupancy in 1977	Percentage Change in 10 Year Period 1967–1977			
			No. of Discharges	No. on Waiting List	No. of Available Staffed Beds	Throughput
General Surgery	Over 100,000	73.6	+8.1	+1.3	−9.2	+19.4
General Medicine		83.6	+27.5	−62.4	−6.4	+36.3
Gynaecology	Between 35,000 and 60,000	69.1	+12.0	−30.0	−0.5	+12.7
Orthopaedic Surgery		76.1	+16.5	+111.3	+4.1	+11.6
Paediatric Medicine		62.7	+36.5	−63.3	+1.2	+35.1
ENT Surgery		58.5	−16.8	−33.2	−12.4	−5.0
Ophthalmology	Around 15,000	63.6	+13.0	+11.0	−3.8	+12.0
Urology		75.7	+79.6	+106.8	+19.2	+50.4
Paediatric Surgery		63.9	−32.7	−24.1	−41.2	+14.3
Chest Medicine	10,000 and below	73.0	+53.2	Negligible List	+13.7	+34.7
Dermatology		73.0	+12.0	−51.2	−7.0	+20.3
Dental Surgery		70.9	+84.2	+3.8	+30.2	+41.4
All-In-patients	508,226 in 1967 575,179 in 1972 521,338 in 1977	73.4	+2.6	+3.3	−17.1	+23.9

Source: Scottish Health Statistics 1977, Table 6.2, Information Services Division.

groups but there has been a massive increase in the number of new attendances per 1,000 population at accident and emergency departments–from 129.1 to 174.0 (34.8 per cent). Another area where there has been a very substantial increase is in the actual numbers of new out-patient attendances for sexually transmitted diseases which rose by 118 per cent from 13,504 to 29,426 between 1967 and 1977.

II.30 From an examination of the trends over the periods covered above, there is in general no evidence that demand for acute services will decrease in the future. The National Medical Consultative Committee pointed to changes in the demand for certain services brought about by new developments in medical techniques and also by epidemiological changes. They have mentioned in particular developments in cardiac surgery (specifically in the pacemaker services), in joint replacement surgery, in urological work including renal transplant surgery and in oncology services; while epidemiological changes included increases in ischaemic heart disease, cancer, sexually transmitted diseases and accidental injuries.

II.31 From a demographic viewpoint, it might be expected that increasing numbers of the elderly in the population will result in a considerable increase in the overall demand for acute hospital services in the future. The age group 75 and over is expected to increase by about 23.5 per cent by 1991, but the 65–74 age group is likely to decrease by 7 per cent over the same period. Within the age group 16–64, the numbers of those aged 45–64 are expected to decrease and those aged 16–44 to increase. The latter group makes the lowest demand upon adult acute hospital services. These population changes will have effects on the demand for acute services which will offset one another to some extent but lead in general to a net increase in demand. An examination has been made of possible effects on the major specialties, viz general medicine, general surgery, orthopaedic surgery, chest medicine, urology and gynaecology, by assuming for the projected 1991 population the same rate of acute bed usage and mean duration of stay for each age group as in 1977, and by examining trends in use over recent years. It appears from this that the increase in total acute bed use in 1991 caused by demographic change will be around 4 per cent on average. The increasing trend in bed-use in most specialties by the age group 75 and over is largely offset by the falling trend for the 65–74 age group; orthopaedics, however, appears to be an exception and the bed-use rate may well continue to rise.

II.32 The overall effect of these changes and trends is to produce a gradual increase in demand associated with some change in the pattern of that demand. There have been decreases in demand in some specialties, principally ear nose and throat (ENT) surgery, but the National Medical Consultative

Committee have indicated that the decrease in tonsil and adenoid operations has permitted ENT surgeons to expand into the growth areas of micro-surgery of the ear and larynx and surgery of malignant tumours of the head and neck. Nevertheless, fewer beds may be required and there could be some release of resources from this specialty. The National Medical Consultative Committee have also suggested that some economies should be possible in the field of respiratory disease, associated with a reduction in smoking brought about by increased health education. The latter also should result in a decrease in chronic bronchitis and lung cancer and there may also be ancillary benefits in reduced coronary artery disease. Savings could also be produced by some rationalisation of the accident and emergency services. Some studies to this end are already in progress. Both the National Medical Consultative Com-mittee and the National Nursing and Midwifery Consultative Committee were of the opinion that considerable savings could be achieved in the cost of drugs, and examination of the use of hospital formularies or drug audits were suggested. Reference was also made to possible savings in the use currently made of radiological and laboratory investigations by existing users. While these savings should be possible with greater discrimination in the use of laboratory services, we recognise that they may be offset by new health care developments requiring laboratory support. Examination of the use made of anaesthetics in the acute services might enable better use to be made of anaesthetic manpower, provide better services and make posts in anaesthetics more attractive. Economies in all these areas would assist the development of priority areas of the acute services.

II.33 If progress in health care is to be maintained, expansion of certain areas of the acute hospital services must take place. We take the view that there is scope for improvement of the efficiency of services and for redistribu-tion of resources. For example, the increase in annual throughput of patients in the past 10 years has been brought about principally by a decrease in the average length of stay in hospital. Variations in the average duration of stay between different hospitals for patients with similar conditions, although in some cases caused by the uneven availability of beds to which patients can be transferred or lack of community facilities, suggest that further decrease is possible. Operational measures such as the introduction, where appropriate, of short stay or day bed facilities or improvement in the provision of diag-nostic or curative support services may help to shorten lengths of stay. Better rehabilitation facilities will also enable patients to be discharged earlier. Clinical divisions and individual clinicians should be encouraged to review their own practices in this area. In this context, we welcome the interest currently being shown by the medical profession in medical audit (which is supported by the Royal Commission on the NHS–paragraph 12.56).

II.34 The other component of throughput, namely average turnover interval (ie the time spent between a patient being discharged and the bed being re-occupied), has been reduced by 7.1 per cent during the past 10 years compared with a 22.6 per cent reduction in duration of stay. Review of hospital and clinical managerial practices, including consideration of an increased degree of flexibility in the use of beds between specialties, may lead to a further decrease.

II.35 The National Medical Consultative Committee and the National Nursing and Midwifery Consultative Committee both draw attention to the problem of beds in acute hospitals occupied by elderly patients who would be more suitably located in long-stay hospitals, or in community facilities, if these were available. In certain cases consultation with experienced geriatricians, who can mobilise the relevant community services more rapidly, can help to relieve the situation. We hope that implementation of our recommendations on priorities will lead to a steady improvement, although this is likely to be spread over a number of years. It must be borne in mind, however, that even if the problem of long-term occupation of beds by the elderly is resolved, there will continue to be a substantial number of beds occupied by elderly patients requiring acute treatment.

II.36 We obtained a rough estimate of the broad financial effect of the various proposals for the acute services and we consider that, while developments on the lines of the priorities suggested by the National Medical Consultative Committee are desirable, these will need to be financed principally by savings within the acute sector. We are aware that over Scotland as a whole there are more beds in the acute (District General Hospital) specialties than are allowed for in the current target ratio of 2.5 beds per 1,000 population (3.0 in those areas which provide teaching facilities for medical schools and act as reference centres).[1] We consider that some health boards must therefore look into the possibility of effecting savings by a reduction in the number of acute beds. (Appendix 1 indicates the broad approximations used to obtain an estimate of savings that might possibly be found throughout Scotland by reducing the total number of acute beds and using them more intensively.) We recognise that achievement of a reduction in acute beds will depend in part on the expansion of geriatric facilities, and in part on the improvements in hospital and clinical management efficiency already discussed. Also, as suggested by the National Consultative Committees, further savings could be effected by the introduction of hospital formularies for drugs, by rationalisation of accident and emergency services and by more discrimination in the use

---

[1]Hospital Plan for Scotland. HMSO 1962.

made of radiodiagnostic and laboratory services by existing users: although in the latter case there may be some offset due to the development of new health care techniques.

II.37 We realise that implementation of the proposal to reduce the number of acute beds may present health boards with considerable difficulties, and Ministerial support will be essential if it is to be carried out, since there will often be strong local pressure to retain facilities in their existing form.

II.38 An important recurring theme in the National Medical Consultative Committee report concerned the problems arising from the introduction of new and sophisticated therapeutic and diagnostic procedures. Such services, which are usually costly, should only be developed in centres where patient demand can be sufficiently concentrated to justify the investment of resources and to maintain at high level the professional skills involved.

II.39 Cardiac surgery is an example of such a centrally funded service in which the decision has already been taken to implement the recommendations of the Cardiac Surgery Programme Planning Group for expansion of services and this commitment has to be accepted. We would, however, suggest that, in the light of the current financial situation, *consideration may need to be given to a slowing down of the rate at which these services are to be developed.* Central funding means that a service is being given overriding priority. Therefore future proposals of this kind should be closely examined in the light of our recommendations on priorities.

II.40 We consider that the developments which should be financed from savings in the acute services as a whole are those proposed by the National Medical Consultative Committee and mentioned in paragraph II.30 above.

(C) CLIENT GROUPS

(i) Maternity and neo-natal services

II.41 Maternity services are provided by general practitioners, obstetricians and midwives, the tasks undertaken by these groups being related to the risk of complications during pregnancy or at birth. Ninety-nine per cent of births now take place in hospital and, in consequence, the number of community-based midwives has fallen sharply. Their work now centres on ante-natal and post-natal care, family planning and parentcraft teaching rather than on deliveries. The general practitioner remains the first point of contact for the pregnant woman.

II.42 The number of maternal deaths has remained at around 0.2 per 1,000 births over the decade to 1977. Increased access to specialist facilities with improvements in ante-natal screening has contributed towards a fairly steady decline in the perinatal mortality rate and a reduction in the prevalence of handicap in the population. Nevertheless the perinatal mortality rate (19.3 per 1,000 total births in 1977) is still high by international standards and the social class differential persists. *The main objectives of the maternity services must be to reduce both the total rate and the class differential,* while at the same time improving care of the mother. A Joint Working Party set up by the National Medical Consultative Committee has recently produced a report on Standards of Perinatal Care and suggested measures for improving them. Some of the report's recommendations have significant financial implications but many, ie those concerned with improvements in professional practice, inter-professional cooperation and local arrangements for the provision of services, do not; *and we recommend that the Joint Working Party's report's recommendations on organisation and professional practice should be implemented.* Similar improvements could be made in neo-natal services without incurring substantial expenditure, particularly in relation to special and intensive care, which would increase infants' chances of survival and reduce the prevalence of long-term handicap. *These improvements in neo-natal care should also be implemented We also support the advice of the NMCC Working Party on Maternal Serum Alphafetoprotein Screening Programme that such screening should be made available routinely to all expectant mothers in Scotland.*

II.43 Admittedly not all causes of perinatal mortality are capable of being reduced by medical intervention; some are environmental and we note the higher than average perinatal mortality rates in areas with large pockets of multiple deprivation. However, even where there are adverse environmental circumstances, further improvements in perinatal mortality could be achieved by better utilisation of neo-natal and ante-natal services. Neo-natal services, particularly those involving special and intensive care, have major implications in terms of both infant survival and long-term handicap: priority should be given to developments in these areas. Late booking or non-attendance at ante-natal clinics should be tackled by improving access to ante-natal clinics (including more convenient opening hours and the siting of clinics nearer to users) and by health education. Already midwives and health visitors are paying more ante-natal and post-natal domiciliary visits to those most at risk, and this trend should be continued. The above considerations suggest that *the uptake of ante-natal services should be improved by encouraging earlier ante-natal attendances by all practicable means and that the visiting of mothers at risk by midwives and health visitors should be extended.* It has been mooted that, in the light of experience abroad, there could be advantage in giving a positive incentive to mothers to attend in early pregnancy, for example, by making the maternity grant payable in whole or in part on first attendance.

II.44 In 1977, 79 per cent of all obstetric beds were in specialist units and this proportion has been gradually increasing in recent years as the number of general practitioner (GP) beds has fallen. Since 1973 the continuing reduction in the number of in-patients discharged from GP beds has been accompanied by a gradual increase in those discharged from specialist beds, which may indicate that the latter are now being used for cases which might previously have been admitted to GP units. The percentage occupancy of specialist beds has risen slightly between 1974 and 1977 to 73.2 per cent while that for GP beds has continued to fall to just under 30 per cent in 1977.

II.45 Increasing awareness of the risks of prematurity, improvements in ante-natal screening techniques and increasing demands on hospital ante-natal clinics have led to a steady increase in ante-natal admissions to specialist beds during the past decade. Despite the fall in the birth rate of some 36 per cent, the number of patients discharged from specialist beds has dropped by only 8 per cent compared with a fall of 40 per cent for GP beds. The average length of stay has been declining (to 7 days in 1977) partly because of the changing balance between admissions for confinements and for ante-natal and post-natal care.

II.46 We consider that the existing maternity beds will be adequate to cope with the projected increase in the number of births in the 1980s. The present number of beds could cope with a greater number of births as occupancy rates are relatively low, especially in GP units. Moreover, while it is expected that the current clinical practice of admitting certain patients for ante-natal screening and care will be maintained, there may be scope for further reduction in post-natal stays. *It ought to be possible to reduce the mean stay for all purposes to six days, and the implementation of this measure offers the greatest scope for savings.* A comparison is made in Table II.2 between the current number of obstetric beds (2,874) and the number of beds required to meet the demand in the peak year for births (1988/89) for each of the variant birth projections discussed in Chapter I. On the basis of the 1977 births/discharges ratio, and of alternative assumptions concerning mean stay and percentage occupancy rates, the births peak could be accommodated within the 1977 total number of beds under any central births projection if a mean stay of six

24

Table II.2 Surplus (+) or Deficiency (−) of beds compared with 1977 total of obstetric beds (2,874)* at births peak in 1988/89

Variant births Projection	Mean stay=7 days		Mean stay=6 days	
	Occupancy rate =80%	Occupancy rate =74%	Occupancy rate =80%	Occupancy rate =74%
High (1976 based)	−664	−951	−159	−405
Central (1976 based)	−352	−613	+109	−115
Low (1976 based)	+112	−112	+507	+315
Central (1977 based)	−301	−559	+152	−68

*Including both specialist (2,272) and GP (602) beds.

Sources: Scottish Health Statistics 1977.
　　　　Table 6.2, ISD.
　　　　Registrar General (Scotland).

days and an occupancy rate of 80 per cent were both achieved. (See Table II.2). If the 1976 based low population forecast proved correct, then the present number of beds would be sufficient if the mean stay of six days was achieved even if the occupancy rate was only 74 per cent; or alternatively if an 80 per cent occupancy rate was achieved with no improvement in mean stay. In all other cases additional beds would be required, and there is therefore a clear case for improving utilisation.

II.47 Further rationalisation might involve closing under-used beds where there are insufficient numbers of births per annum to maintain medical and nursing skills. Such rationalisation by closure or transfer of maternity beds, while perhaps less convenient for the patient, is likely to improve standards of care. Therefore we recommend that *the utilisation of existing maternity in-patient facilities should be improved by closing under-used beds or transferring them to other uses*.

(ii) **Child health**

II.48 Health services for children are provided in the community by the general practitioner, by other members of the primary care team, in particular the health visitor, and by the school health service. Within the hospital service, a wide variety of specialties and disciplines is engaged to varying degrees in the diagnosis, assessment, care and treatment of children. Principal among these are the specialties of medical and surgical paediatrics and of child psychiatry, which are specifically orientated towards the needs of the sick child.

II.49 There has been a steady decrease in the child population over the past decade (see Chapter I(C)). The effect of this is most noticeable in the workload of health visitors, in that visits to pre-school children accounted for only 56 per cent of their caseload in 1977 compared with over 71 per cent in 1967. The average number of visits paid to each child, however, has altered very little. Similarly the number of school entrants examined by the school health service has dropped over 15 per cent between 1970 and 1977, although leavers examined have increased. As noted in paragraph I.9, the 5–15 age group will continue to decline in numbers between now and 1986, and this might be seen as justifying a reduction in resources devoted to community child health services. However the numbers of pre-school children will be greater in 1986 than in 1977, and we have been impressed by the need for the development of new services highlighted in the reports of the Child Health Programme Planning Group. Its report on vulnerable families has been taken account of in our own proposals for improving services to multiply deprived households in Chapter IV. It draws attention to the need for an expansion in the number of health visitors to remedy local deficiencies and to meet the needs of areas of social deprivation.

II.50 The Programme Planning Group's report on health services for children at school includes proposals for comprehensive health surveillance of children of school age following on pre-school health surveillance on the lines of the Court Report.[1] The main proposals are for the replacement of the present school leaver's examination (which in some cases is still carried out as a universal procedure) with a selective examination, the introduction of annual nurse/pupil interviews and the extension of the school health service to pre-school children in playgroups, day nurseries and nursery schools. The report's section on children with handicap proposes multidisciplinary assessment of children with handicap (of all ages), shared between health and education services and in close collaboration with social work services. We acknowledge the importance of surveillance measures, but their full implementation would be very costly, and the needs of children must be weighed against those of other groups, particularly the expanding over 75 population. We

---

[1]Fit for the Future: The Report of the Committee on Child Health Services. HMSO Cmnd. 6684, 1976.

would be reluctant to recommend the implementation of the Child Health Programme Planning Group's surveillance proposals, if this were to lead to an increase in the resources devoted to child health, before these proposals had been fully evaluated in pilot projects. *We think that as and when resources are freed by the reduction in the school population, the surveillance measures recommended by the Child Health Programme Planning Group report should be evaluated by the establishment of pilot projects.* The position should be reviewed in the next planning round in the light of this evaluation.

II.51 More emphasis should be laid on the prevention of childhood illness, with the care and treatment of children increasingly being carried out in the community. Particular attention should be paid to the needs of children in areas of multiple deprivation. Vaccination and immunisation have contributed substantially to the reduced incidence of infectious disease in children, although current rates of uptake are not satisfactory. The acceptance rate for pertussis (whooping cough) has in fact declined from 78 per cent to 55 per cent during the period 1970 to 1977, mainly because of unfavourable publicity about the possibilities of vaccine damage. However, the Joint Committee on Vaccination and Immunisation reviewed the evidence in 1977 and concluded that, provided attention is paid to contra-indications to vaccination, the benefits of protection far outweigh any risk of side effects. The acceptance rate for measles has increased to about 50 per cent of the 3-year old population but it still falls far below the target level of 85–90 per cent recommended by the Department in 1976. The acceptance rate for rubella (German measles) had increased to 82.5 per cent of 14-year old girls in 1977, but the aim is to achieve a 95 per cent uptake of rubella vaccination as soon as possible. *Health education measures aimed at achieving an adequate uptake of these services should be increased.*

II.52 Despite the fall in the child population, the number of new medical paediatric out-patients has remained constant while in some specialties, eg in child psychiatry and accident and emergency, the number of new out-patients has actually increased over the last few years. The National Medical Consultative Committee's Report on the Study of Acute Hospital Services suggests that many children admitted to hospital for investigations could be dealt with on an out-patient basis if adequate facilities were available. The report recommends that better out-patient facilities, including day beds, should be provided and that paediatric out-patient facilities should be made more widely available in hospitals and health centres. This development would reduce the need for expensive in-patient facilities. We agree that *out-patient facilities be extended to peripheral hospitals and health centres, and that there should be increased provision of day beds.*

II.53 As regards in-patient services, discharges of children from non-psychiatric hospitals have declined by almost 12 per cent over the last 10 years and the numbers of children admitted to, and resident in, mental handicap and mental illness hospitals have also been decreasing. Owing mainly to a fall in the average length of stay, occupancy rates for both medical and surgical paediatric beds have fallen, despite a considerable reduction (from 581 to 346) in staffed surgical paediatric beds. The proportion of children accommodated in children's hospitals and paediatric units rather than in adult wards has increased over the decade from 41.1 per cent to 50.1 per cent of the total, consolidating the trend noted in 'Towards an Integrated Child Health Service'.[1] The period between 1970 and 1977 has also seen increases in the number of consultants in medical paediatrics (from 38 to 58 whole-time equivalent) and little change (from 11 to 10 whole-time equivalent)[2] in the number of consultants in surgical paediatrics. In the future the demand for in-patient services should lessen as the total child population falls. This, together with the trend towards earlier discharge, suggests that some hospital beds could be closed. These closures might be in peripheral units which are too small to meet the needs of children and maintain the skills of medical and nursing staff and such closures should improve the overall quality of service. However, this should not be done until the out-patient facilities recommended above are available to provide services required locally. Subject to that caveat, *paediatric in-patient services should be rationalised with closures of units which are too small to meet the needs of children and maintain the skills of medical and nursing staff.*

II.54 It has been necessary to consider the various aspects of the child health services separately, particularly for the purpose of cost calculations; but we would like to emphasise that the child health services should be regarded as a unity, as described in the Brotherston Report. Child health care will benefit not only from the improvements in prevention, health surveillance and vaccination and immunisation discussed in paragraphs II.50–51, but also from the implementation of objectives proposed for other programmes in this report, for example in relation to handicap and multiple deprivation. Therefore while some child health services, eg hospital paediatrics, may be expected to decline as a result of the falling child population, it will be seen that considerable importance is being given to child health as a whole in this report.

---

[1]Towards an Integrated Child Health Service. HMSO 1973.
[2]And even this apparent fall is misleading, since the 1977 figure would have been 11 except for a temporary vacancy at the census date.

(iii) Care of the elderly

II.55 The main determinant of need for services for the elderly is the size and composition of the population aged 65 and over and in particular the age group 75 and over. Other factors affecting need include social circumstances and levels of morbidity and disability, both physical and mental, which increase with advancing age. The number of people aged 65 and over is expected to increase by 3.8 per cent to just over 732,000 by 1991. The age structure of the group is likely to change considerably with a reduction of 6.9 per cent projected in the 65–74 age group and an increase of 23.5 per cent in the age group 75 and over, and this will increase the demand for both health and social work services.

II.56 The increase in numbers of the very elderly means that there is likely to be an increased demand for residential care both in hospital and in local authority homes. The vast majority of the elderly, however, will continue to live in their own homes, though some will attend day hospitals, and elderly persons who become ill or disabled will require rehabilitation so that they can lead as independent a life as possible. In this respect paramedical therapeutic services such as physiotherapy and chiropody must be made more readily available in the community. Local authority services, in particular social work services, and the primary care and other community health services will have to meet an increasing demand from the elderly living in the community. A policy of caring for more old people in the community rather than in hospital can succeed only if local authorities and voluntary agencies provide the necessary social work and housing services. Conversely, if local authorities fail to make the necessary provision for financial or other reasons, a much greater load will fall on the health services. *The overall objective should be to prevent inappropriate admissions to long-stay hospital accommodation by means of increased emphasis on care and support of the elderly in the community.*

II.57 Research in progress suggests that many elderly persons with short-term illness who are at present admitted to acute medical wards could, if 'augmented home care' were made available, be more effectively treated in their own homes. This hospital-at-home concept, in which the resources of the hospital are brought to the sick elderly person in his or her own home, has been introduced in England in the Medway Health District while a scheme in Peterborough has been sponsored by the Sainsbury Trust. This innovation still requires to be evaluated both in respect of the outcome of treatment and the ratio of costs to benefits. However this concept, if successful, would prevent some acute hospital admissions which can in turn lead to an elderly person requiring longer-term care. *We therefore recommend that these schemes should be studied carefully with a view to introducing them if the current evaluation is satisfactory.*

II.58 The target level for provision of geriatric beds in hospitals is at present linked to the number of people 65 and over at a rate of 15 beds per 1,000 population over 65. However, the Programme Planning Group on Care of the Elderly in Scotland recommended that the provision of beds and places should be based on the number aged 75 and over. We agree with that view, since it is the over 75 rather than the over 65 population which requires long-term care. We think that *the future planning of geriatric beds should be related to the 75 and over age group, and that the PPG's proposed basic minimum ratio of 40 beds per 1,000 population aged 75 or over seems reasonable.* The 1981 requirement would be 10,900 beds, compared with the 1977 total of 10,126,[1] whether the over 65 or the over 75 ratio is used. However, in 1986 the over 75 ratio would give a target of 11,900 beds, while a ratio related to the over 65 population would leave the target at 10,900. Around 650 extra beds are projected under the major and ordinary building programmes by 1986. This would still leave a shortfall at that date, though more beds are included in the building programme for completion later.

II.59 Geriatric hospital provision cannot be considered in isolation, since the demand for hospital beds depends on the provision made in the community, including sheltered and amenity housing as well as residential homes. In March 1976 in Scotland as a whole there were some 9,000 residential places for the elderly in local authority homes and 5,000 places in voluntary homes, giving a total rate of 19.9 places per 1,000 persons over 65 compared with the present target rate of 25 places. As at 30 April 1978, the total number of special housing places completed, under construction or approved awaiting start was 11,300 for sheltered housing and 6,200 for amenity housing. These are well short of the Programme Planning Group's targets of 50 places in sheltered housing and 100 places in amenity housing per 1,000 people over 65. There is clearly a need to expand community as well as hospital provision and, in view of the links between the two types of provision, *health boards should cooperate closely with local authorities in drawing up plans for residential provision for the elderly which would achieve overall a proper balance between hospital and community care.*

II.60 The report of the Programme Planning Group on Care of the Elderly has recommended a ratio of two geriatric day hospital places per 1,000 population aged 65 and over. Applying this rate to the 1977 population

---

[1]There were also around 160 GP long-stay beds in 1977.

produces a current requirement of 1,410 day places, which would rise to 1,464 by 1991. No accurate data on the level of current provision are available but such information as can be obtained suggests a considerable shortfall. While *the ratio of two geriatric day hospital places per 1,000 population aged 65 and over recommended by the Programme Planning Group seems reasonable to us as a target to aim for*, we are aware that there are difficulties over the supply of transport essential for the running of day hospitals (see Appendix 2, paragraphs 26–27).

(iv) **Elderly with mental disability**

II.61 The number of elderly residents (aged 65 and over) in mental illness hospitals has risen from just over 7,800 in 1964 (then 40 per cent of all residents[1]) to almost 9,200 in 1977 (53 per cent of all residents). The projected increase in the general population of those aged 75 and over–the group most susceptible to mental illness–makes improvement in services for the elderly with mental disability a matter of priority. Most of this group suffer from dementia.

II.62 The Report on Services for the Elderly with Mental Disability in Scotland[2] has estimated that, in addition to the 3,000 or so patients suffering from dementia who are currently accommodated in mental hospitals, about 750 demented patients are inappropriately located in acute hospitals or geriatric hospitals and a further 1,250 such patients requiring considerable nursing care are at present located in local authority residential homes and voluntary homes. In addition, a sizeable number of elderly people in the community have unmet needs and require hospital care. The report, therefore, recommends hospital provision for old people with dementia of 10 beds per 1,000 population aged 65 and over, ie, 7,050 beds rising to 7,300 in 1991, half of which would be in small to medium units, called 'continuing care' units, in close proximity to the community they served. These units would be provided in single storey buildings of 40–60 beds (two or three 20-bed units) containing single or four-bed rooms and with separate day activity areas providing both for the residents and day patients. They would have an essentially domestic atmosphere and be staffed mainly by nursing assistants with qualified nurse

---

[1]A 'resident' in this context is a patient in hospital on 31 December in a particular year.
[2]SHHD and SED Services for the Elderly with Mental Disability in Scotland: A Report by a Programme Planning Group of the Scottish Health Service Planning Council and the Advisory Council on Social Work [Chairman: Dr G. C. Timbury] Edinburgh, HMSO 1979.

supervision. We recognise that care of the elderly with mental disability must have a high priority, but the financial and other resources required to meet the ratio of 10 beds per 1,000 persons over 65 would be very large. 4,000 new beds and 1,500 replacement beds, together with over 900 extra nursing staff, would be needed to meet this ratio by 1986. Therefore, while the target of *10 beds per 1,000 people over 65 for the elderly with dementia* may be justifiable, it seems unlikely that this target could be attained for some time (see Chapter VI). The best hope for making progress towards the target, at reasonable cost, may lie with adapting existing units which are no longer required for their present purpose.

II.63 Only 11 out of the 34 health districts in Scotland provide special day facilities for psychiatric conditions in the elderly. The Timbury Report *suggests a provision of day hospital places of 2.5 per 1,000 persons aged 65 and over and suggests that the level of provision might need to be increased to 3 per 1,000 to take into account the rising proportion of those aged 75 and over. If this suggestion were adopted, a total of 2,200 day places would be required by 1991.*

(v) Mental illness

II.64 A substantial proportion of mental illness is dealt with in the community by the primary health care services, voluntary agencies, and the local authority social work services. The extent to which these services can expand their capacity to enable more patients to be treated in the community rather than in hospital will be a major factor in determining the balance to be struck within the NHS between treatment by the primary care team and by the specialist services. Much will depend on what progress is made in the education of health workers, voluntary workers and the wider community in the management of psychiatric illness. While the mental illness hospital is still the main base for psychiatry in Scotland, despite the development of psychiatric units in general hospitals, a new level of involvement on the part of the community must be the primary consideration.

II.65 Hospital treatment for the mentally ill (including the elderly with mental disability) is at present provided chiefly in mental illness hospitals and in psychiatric units in general hospitals or in special units for children and adolescents. Some mentally ill patients are also accommodated at the State Hospital, Carstairs. Nevertheless, while hospitals will continue to play a major role, it should be the general policy to care for patients as far as possible within the community, either in their own homes or in conditions approximating as nearly as possible to their own homes. In this respect rehabilitation and resettlement are important and involve contact and co-operation with employment services and with the authorities responsible for such services as sheltered workshops, housing and hostel accommodation. Both day hospitals and day centres, the latter essentially a social work provision receiving support from the mental health team, have important and complementary roles to play in maintaining patients within the community and in creating a harmonious balance between hospital and community care. *The main objective, as indicated to us by the Mental Illness Subcommittee of the Mental Disorder Programme Planning Group, should be to work towards a community based service for mental illness by means of a joint planning approach by the health service and local authorities in liaison with voluntary agencies.*

II.66 Some progress towards this aim has already been made. Between 1965 and 1977, the number of admissions to mental illness hospitals and psychiatric units has risen by some 23 per cent from 19,823 to 24,459. Discharges have followed a very similar pattern. In contrast the number of residents[1] has declined by 13 per cent from 19,984 to 17,380. This would seem to indicate an increased demand for hospital psychiatric services offset by a higher turnover rate and a decrease in the number of occupied beds. The proportion of patients discharged to their homes rose from 41 per cent to 73 per cent between 1965 and 1970, though little change has occurred since then.

II.67 Females are considerably more likely to be admitted to a mental illness hospital than males; in 1977 there were nearly 500 female admissions per 100,000 population compared with just over 440 admissions for males. Admissions related to alcoholism have increased from 25 per cent to 35 per cent of all male admissions and for female admissions from 4 per cent to over 9 per cent. Action to deal with the growing problem of alcoholism is considered in Chapter V. Cases of drug dependence, though relatively few, have doubled in numbers since 1965 for male admissions but almost halved for females. Admissions for depression, always consistently higher for females than for males, have shown a steady decline for both sexes, perhaps indicating increasing opportunities for treating such cases outwith hospital.

II.68 With regard to child and adolescent mental health,[2] the Mental Disorder Programme Planning Group has recommended to our Working Party

---

[1] A 'resident' in this context is a patient in hospital on 31 December in a particular year.
[2] The Working Group on Child and Adolescent Mental Health, under the chairmanship of Professor Elizabeth M. Mapstone, will report more fully in due course.

that, among other developments, the aim should be to provide over the next decade $1\frac{1}{2}$ whole-time equivalent child and adolescent psychiatrists per 200,000 total population. This would involve an increase from the 1977 total of 26 whole-time equivalent to 39 whole-time equivalent. The specialist psychiatric services for children and adolescents in Scotland are unevenly distributed and require systematic development, the paramount need being for a more multi-disciplinary team approach involving, amongst others, psychiatrists, nurses, clinical psychologists, social workers and voluntary personnel.

(vi) Mental handicap

II.69 The great majority of the mentally handicapped live at home. In addition to requiring primary health care services, they also require assessment services, social work services, education services, and hospital and specialist services. Hospital services for the mentally handicapped cater for the most severely disabled of the mentally handicapped population, and account for most of the NHS expenditure on this client group. Continued improvements in hospital and community services for the mentally handicapped were accorded priority in 'The Way Ahead'.

II.70 Estimates of the prevalence of mental handicap in the Scottish population were included in the 1972 joint SHHD/SED Memorandum 'Services for the Mentally Handicapped'[1] and the 1979 Report 'A Better Life'[2] by a sub-committee of the Mental Disorder Programme Planning Group. There is a substantial difference between the two estimates, arising from the PPG's view that the prevalence rate for adults with moderate/severe handicap is 3.0 per 1,000 instead of the earlier Report's estimate of 2.0 per 1,000. This view was reached partly on the grounds that mentally handicapped persons are now living longer. Although the incidence of handicap is not expected to increase and the total number of mentally handicapped persons will fall by 1986 as a result of expected population changes, the Report points out that the total number of persons with moderate or severe handicap will not change. Further small reductions in prevalence might be obtained by advances in ante-natal care and screening of women in early pregnancy.

---

[1] SHHD, SED Services for the Mentally Handicapped. Edinburgh, HMSO 1972.
[2] SHHD, SED A Better Life: Services for the Mentally Handicapped in Scotland: A Report by a Programme Planning Group of the Scottish Health Service Planning Council and the Advisory Council on Social Work [Chairman: Mr D. A. Peters] Edinburgh, HMSO 1979.

II.71 In 1977 there were 1.55 mentally handicapped residents in hospital (including those in mental illness hospitals) per 1,000 population, and if those on the waiting list are added to give an estimate of the total demand for hospital places the ratio would rise to 1.64. By contrast the ratio of residents in community accommodation to population is only 0.18 per 1,000. The Mental Disorder Programme Planning Group stated that, while an overall ratio of 1.8 hospital beds and residential places per 1,000 population was a reasonable interim target figure, a shift from hospital to community accommodation was required to give 1.2 hospital beds and 0.6 community places per 1,000 population. It also suggested this balance might be further altered in the future in favour of increased community provision.

II.72 In arriving at its recommended bed ratio, the PPG estimated that the number of mentally handicapped in-patients could be reduced by a quarter as community provision expanded. However, a major constraint on any massive reduction in the number of existing hospital residents is that the majority, many of whom are elderly, have been in hospital for a very long time and would find it difficult to adapt to life outside. There is more scope for preventing long lengths of stay for new admissions by increasing support for the mentally handicapped and their families in the community, by providing day care and out-patient services and, wherever possible, by admitting patients for short periods for assessment or training only. Support in the community would require the assistance of social work (and education) services. In order *to bring about a shift of emphasis from hospital to community care with the eventual aim of reducing hospital beds to 1.2 per 1,000 population, action should be taken in association with local authorities to prevent inappropriate admissions to hospitals.*

II.73 Certain mental handicap hospitals are badly sited in relation to the population they serve, with 40 per cent of beds being concentrated in the two largest hospitals, whose catchment areas are extensive. *Large hospitals should be reduced in size and smaller units provided in reasonable proximity to the population they serve.* Since this is likely to take many years, there is need in the meantime for the upgrading of certain hospitals; *the process of upgrading standards of accommodation in existing mental handicap hospitals should be continued.* It would not seem reasonable to delay such improvements until a decision has been reached on the Jay Report's recommendation for small family-type homes, which may have relatively long-term implications.

II.74 A major problem in achieving a redistribution of beds and improvements in staff ratios will be the availability of staff locally. There is already a shortage of medical staff, nursing staff (particularly qualified nursing staff) and paramedical staff in mental handicap hospitals and recruitment difficulties are being experienced. The proposals of the Jay Report for training of mental handicap care staff to be within the social services framework, and for the number of staff to be doubled, would, if implemented, be of a radical nature. The implications for recruitment in several fields are considerable and the suggestion of changes of this kind may already be making recruitment of mental handicap nurses more difficult. Consultant posts in mental handicap are very difficult to fill.

(vii) Physically handicapped

Numbers of handicapped

II.75 Estimates of the numbers of physically handicapped in Scotland[1] based on the 1971 Harris Report[2] showed that there were approximately 274,000 handicapped persons over the age of 16 living in private households. It has also been estimated that in a population of 10,000, 29 persons would be very severely handicapped (three-quarters being aged over 65), 180 would be severely or appreciably handicapped and 359 would have a handicap of little significance.

Causes of handicap

II.76 The Harris report showed that the most important cause of very severe disability is disease of the central nervous system, 24 per cent of which is caused by stroke. Fifty per cent of severe or appreciable handicap results from disease of the bones or organs of movement, principally arthritis, which is also the commonest cause of minor disability. The report estimated that 25 per cent of all handicapped people aged 16–64 suffered from disease of the bones or organs of movement. While these figures refer to Great Britain as a whole, the Scottish figures are unlikely to be very different.

Prevention of handicap

II.77 Good obstetric care can play a part by reducing the incidence of birth injuries and subsequent handicap, and attendance at ante-natal clinics should

[1]Mrs V. Carstairs. Health Bulletin. Volume XXX No. 2, April 1972.
[2]Handicapped and Impaired in Great Britain. Amelia Harris, 1971.

be encouraged. Immunisation and vaccination will continue to make a significant contribution to prevention of handicap.

Care of the physically handicapped

II.78 Care of the physically handicapped is provided by the primary care team, the hospital service, local authorities and voluntary agencies separately or in collaboration depending upon the level and nature of the disability. According to the form of his disability, the handicapped adult makes varied use of the services offered. However, all surveys have noted the uneven delivery of these various services and, equally, the variable uptake of the services by the handicapped themselves. We think there should be an *overall plan to coordinate the growth and development of services for the physically handicapped.* This plan should (as is the case for other long-term care services) have the general aim of *improving the community services to enable the physically handicapped to live at home wherever possible.*

Young chronic sick

II.79 The physically handicapped living in hospital should be in appropriate accommodation, which for the young chronic sick (ie those under 65 years of age) is, ideally, specialised units staffed by suitably experienced staff. The annual census of young chronic sick accommodated in wards wholly or mainly used for the care of elderly persons, required by the Chronically Sick and Disabled Persons Act 1970, shows that the number of such persons (who are misplaced in terms of the Act) in non-psychiatric hospitals has slowly fallen from 522 in 1973 to 396 in 1977. The total number of young chronic sick in hospital has also been falling, from 1,580 in 1972 to 947 in 1977. *Nevertheless there is a continuing need to ensure that the young chronic sick living in hospital are placed in appropriate accommodation.* The adoption of the recently approved CSA building design guidance for new young chronic sick units will facilitate this.

Rehabilitation

II.80 Problems encountered at present in the provision of rehabilitation programmes and services include a lack of coordination between the various bodies involved and there is a *strong case for improvements in cooperation between all involved in the care of the physically handicapped.* This problem may be aggravated by the fact that there is no current requirement in Scotland for local authorities to maintain registers of handicapped and disabled persons, so that estimates of total numbers of handicapped may not be reliable. *It is of prime importance that those in need of care are identified so that continuing care and support, whether in the community or in hospital, can be provided.*

II.81 There is a need for development of rehabilitation programmes and services for the physically handicapped, including the pre-school and school age child. The Child Health Programme Planning Group has proposed a multi-disciplinary system of assessment of children with handicap (see paragraph II.50) and the Mair[1] Report made a strong recommendation, endorsed by 'The Way Ahead', for the effective development of rehabilitation programmes for the physically handicapped. We think *the NHS should adopt the aim of maintaining and improving services of special importance for the physically handicapped.*

Prosthetics and orthotics

II.82 The National Centre for Training and Education in Prosthetics and Orthotics, established in 1973, has improved standards of training in prosthetics and orthotics and is also active in promoting courses and seminars for groups both within and outside the NHS with an interest in prosthetics and orthotics. One problem in this field is a shortage of skilled shoemakers which could lead to a crisis in the orthopaedic footwear service in five years time and *there is a need to take action now to increase the supply of shoemakers.*

(D) SUPPORT SERVICES

II.83 We considered two main kinds of support services: (i) scientific services; and (ii) the ambulance service. The scientific services, which are now being developed in an orderly way in support of medicine, we subdivided into: diagnostic services–radiodiagnosis, ultrasonography, medical laboratory services; treatment services–blood transfusion service, anaesthetic services; and other clinical support services–medical physics and bio-engineering. We recognised that there are other services which could properly be placed

---

[1] Medical Rehabilitation: The Pattern for the Future. SHHD/Scottish Health Services Council 1972.

in this category, but in view of their heterogeneous nature we did not examine their role in any detail. This is not to deny their importance, however. Nor did we consider in this context such scientific services as radiotherapy, which are provided within specific clinical units, and clinical psychology departments, which are responsible for giving direct health care as well as supplying scientific support services.

II.84 We concluded that as the need for the development of support services is largely determined by the demands made upon them by health care programmes it was not necessary to include in the main body of our report anything other than this brief section. But, to give some indication of what is involved in these support services which we examined, we include at Appendix 2 some notes on each of them.

III   Provision of Resources: Manpower and Finance

Introduction

III.1 Although priorities can, in theory, be considered in isolation from the availability of manpower and financial resources, this does not make good sense. In the following paragraphs of this chapter we review these resources and draw attention to some points which are of importance in our subsequent consideration of priorities. In particular the emphasis being placed on the expansion of community services and on preventive measures will have implications for all health care staff, as well as for related groups, eg social workers and voluntary agencies.

(A)   MANPOWER

(i)   General survey

III.2 The numbers working in the NHS in Scotland are very large; in 1977 there were around 117,000 whole-time equivalent, of whom 3,800 were employed in the Common Services Agency while all the rest were employed by, or were in contract with, health boards. Four-fifths of health board staff were employed in hospitals, though the proportion has fallen slightly in recent years.

III.3 The NHS employs a large number of different manpower groups, many of which are small. Table III.1 shows hospital manpower (whole-time equivalent) in the years 1967-1977 divided into 11 groups; some of these groups, eg professions supplementary to medicine and ancillary staff, are made up of a number of different professions or trades. By far the largest group are nurses, who now account for just over half of all (whole-time equivalent) hospital staff. Ancillary and other staff account for around another one-quarter. Of the remaining nine groups only two, doctors and

Table III.1 Hospital Manpower by Group (WTE) 1967–1977 as at 30 September

Group	1967	1968	1969	1970	1971	1972	1973	1974	1975	1976	1977	Average Increase pa (compound) 1967–77 (%)
1. Medical	3,396	3,546	3,673	3,866	4,080	4,260	4,373	4,417	4,509	4,591	4,714	3.3
2. Dental	91	105	119	138	154	154	160	164	171	171	172	6.6
3. Nursing	34,806	35,183	35,957	37,573	39,938	42,208	43,666	44,642	48,152	48,838	48,577	3.4
4. Pharmacists	197	195	200	214	221	237	234	242	282	313	314	4.8
5. Opticians	15	15	16	21	21	23	21	21	19	24	20	2.9
6. Professions Supplementary to Medicine*	1,594	1,575	1,640	1,725	1,811	1,826	1,858	1,900	2,210	2,254	2,293	3.7
7. Scientists	129	144	153	174	182	231	237	254	321	347	381	11.4
8. Technical	1,916	2,046	2,167	2,339	2,503	2,656	2,833	2,747	3,108	3,199	3,330	5.7
9. Works†	1,940	2,001	1,974	2,183	2,248	2,292	2,319	2,416	2,622	2,692	2,666	3.2
10. Ancillary and others	22,397	22,670	22,878	23,255	23,735	24,152	24,226	25,364	25,707	25,944	25,994	1.5
11. Administrative and Clerical	3,172	3,395	3,648	3,860	4,167	4,506	4,952	5,555	5,819	6,252	6,132	6.8
All Groups	69,653	70,875	72,425	75,348	79,060	82,545	84,879	87,722	92,920	94,625	94,593	3.1

Source: ISD.

*Includes Speech Therapists.
†Includes Maintenance Craftsmen and Tradesmen.

administrative and clerical staff, each make up more than 5 per cent of the total. While total numbers of staff have been growing fairly rapidly–3.1 per cent per annum (compound) on average between 1967 and 1977–some groups have grown much more rapidly than others. The most rapid growth rates were recorded for scientists and technicians, dentists, and administrative and clerical staff. The one group to grow much more slowly than average was ancillary and other staff (Table III.1).

III.4 Reliable and comprehensive information for NHS manpower based outwith hospitals (including community health service staff and headquarters etc staff) is available only since 1974. The available figures (which exclude pharmacists) are shown in Table III.2, together with the hospital figures for comparison. Dentists, opticians and pharmacists work mainly in the family practitioner services; and the balance for administrative staff has shifted in the years since 1974 towards the non-hospital sector. All other groups are based mainly in hospitals, particularly nurses. Staff numbers are growing more rapidly in the community than in hospitals (23 per cent between 1974 and 1977 compared with 8 per cent for hospital staff).

III.5 Most NHS staff are women, and the proportion is increasing (though this proportion varies from group to group, tending to be lower for university educated staff, senior posts and traditionally male groups like works staff). In 1977, 79 per cent of all hospital staff (whole-time equivalent) were females; the proportion for staff other than hospital staff was 58 per cent. The increase in the proportion of female staff, who often have domestic commitments, was accompanied in general by an increase in part-time working (though there have been exceptions to this, and the correlation is not precise). The Scottish Health Service, as one of the largest employers of female labour in Scotland and therefore depending on being an attractive employer to women, will have to pay special attention to the needs of female employees. Competition in the female labour market may become fiercer in future because the general pattern of employment is tending towards industries, including service industries, which employ large numbers of women, although this might not be true if high unemployment rates continue. The provision of flexible working hours and opportunities for part-time work may be the best methods of attracting women with domestic commitments. These modes of employ-ment are also useful to the NHS in dealing with peak loads and filling posi-tions where full-time personnel are not required. The provision of creches, and refresher training courses for qualified personnel, eg speech therapists, returning to employment after a break of some years, may encourage women to return to NHS employment.

Table III.2 Manpower by Group and Location 1974–77 (WTE)

Group		1974	1975	1976	1977
1. Medical	Hospital	4,417	4,509	4,591	4,714
	Non-hospital	3,325	3,481	3,530	3,572
	Total	7,742	7,990	8,121	8,286
2. Dental	Hospital	164	171	171	172
	Non-hospital	1,469	1,482	1,508	1,516
	Total	1,633	1,653	1,679	1,688
3. Nursing	Hospital	44,642	48,152	48,838	48,577
	Non-hospital	3,646	4,267	4,435	4,499
	Total	48,288	52,419	53,273	53,076
4. Scientists	Hospital	254	321	347	381
	Non-hospital	111	103	128	135
	Total	365	424	475	516
5. Professions Supplementary to Medicine*	Hospital	1,900	2,210	2,254	2,293
	Non-hospital	255	351	493	450
	Total	2,155	2,561	2,747	2,743
6. Technical	Hospital	2,747	3,108	3,199	3,330
	Non-hospital	708	930	992	1,106
	Total	3,455	4,038	4,191	4,436
7. Works†	Hospital	2,416	2,622	2,692	2,666
	Non-hospital	495	538	568	637
	Total	2,911	3,160	3,260	3,303
8. Administrative and Clerical	Hospital	5,555	5,819	6,252	6,132
	Non-hospital	5,005	6,393	6,436	6,506
	Total	10,560	12,212	12,688	12,638
9. Ancillary and others	Hospital	25,364	25,707	25,944	25,994
	Non-hospital	2,044	2,437	2,845	2,697
	Total	27,408	28,144	28,789	28,691
10. Pharmacists‡	Hospital	242	282	313	314
11. Opticians	Hospital	21	19	24	20
	Non-hospital§	657	642	605	610
	Total	(678)	(661)	(629)	(630)
	Hospital	87,480	92,638	94,601	94,279
All Groups	Non-hospital	17,715	20,624	21,540	21,728
	Total	105,195	113,262	115,852	116,007

Source: ISD.

*Including Speech Therapists.

†Includes maintenance craftsmen and tradesmen.

‡Figures are not available for pharmacists outside hospitals; their numbers were believed to be between 1,200 and 1,300 in 1977.

§Opticians in general practice.

III.6 Three-quarters of all hospital revenue expenditure in 1976/77 was on salaries, and the proportion is rising slowly. Proper control of hospital staffing, therefore, will ensure control of the major part of hospital costs. Conversely, it will be difficult to increase total numbers (whole-time equivalent) of hospital staff more rapidly than total hospital revenue expenditure, unless the average cost per employee declines. And a rapid increase in numbers of any large group, eg nurses, can be achieved only if the growth of other groups is held back; this constraint is less important for small groups, eg scientists, which account for only a small part of wage costs.

III.7 Although information about the proportions of expenditure on community health services which went on staff salaries is not readily available, it seems likely that similar considerations to those outlined in paragraph III.6 apply to them too.

III.8 We now look at current issues and problems relating to key manpower groups, ie doctors, nurses, administrative and clerical staff and paramedical therapeutic staff. (Dental manpower is considered in Chapter II(A)(ii) in the context of Primary Dental Care, in which most dentists are engaged.)

(ii) **Medical manpower**

III.9 Since the market for doctors is a UK one, measures to control the overall demand and supply of doctors can only be taken at a UK level. Moreover, adjustment of the total number of doctors by regulating the intake to medical schools will have very little impact during the period up to 1986. This section concentrates, therefore, on issues on which action can be taken within this timespan in Scotland, ie maldistribution, either geographical or by specialty. (Long-term manpower planning at the UK level has been considered in the health departments' recent paper, 'Medical Manpower – The Next Twenty Years'.[1])

III.10 Geographical maldistribution exists in both general practice and hospital sectors, but is not a significant problem for community medicine. In general practice there have been problems in finding general practitioners for deprived inner city areas, and a few individual boards also have noticeably worse general practitioner/population ratios than others. While financial incentives are already paid to general practitioners to attract them to under-doctored areas, these incentives have been criticised for being insufficiently flexible. A joint working party, whose remit included 'to suggest criteria by which under doctored areas might be identified, and measures which might

---

[1]Health Departments 1978: HMSO.

44

be taken to achieve an adequate number of doctors in such areas', produced an inconclusive report in 1979. The General Medical Services Committee (the official representative body for general practitioners) has subsequently set up a working group to consider the problems further.

III.11 Geographical maldistribution of manpower within the hospital service has long historical roots. This maldistribution has been intensified by such factors as migration from one area to another. In addition the building of new district general hospitals in previously under-provided areas has led to short-term difficulties in the provision of staff, especially in certain specialties, such as anaesthetics.

III.12 The overall position is continuously monitored by the Advisory Committee on Hospital Medical Establishments which comprises Departmental and professional representatives, and which advises the Secretary of State on the creation of all new hospital posts. The SHARE redistribution of revenue monies will encourage boards at present well provided either to reduce or to stabilise their hospital establishment and thus enable the increase of establishments in areas which are at present relatively less well staffed. A general freeze has been imposed on junior staff with a few exceptions such as new district general hospitals and a voluntary freeze on the consultant establishment in Glasgow has been adopted by the Health Board. The Royal Commission on the NHS has recommended that 'the Health Departments should show more determination in enforcing their priorities in the medical staff shortage specialties, if necessary by blocking expansion of other specialties' (paragraph 14.32), and presumably this point will be further examined.

(iii)   **Nursing manpower**

III.13 While the total number (whole-time equivalent) of nurses increased by 29 per cent between 1970 and 1977, from 37,000 to 48,600, the relative rates of increases for unqualified and qualified staff were very different. Qualified staff increased by 28 per cent but numbers of unqualified staff increased by 40 per cent. Moreover, numbers of student and pupil nurses who (together with qualified nurses returning to work) provide the qualified staff of the future increased by only 19 per cent. Within the qualified group the proportion of enrolled nurses rose from 29 per cent to 34 per cent between 1970 and 1977. (It should be noted, however, that changes in conditions of service, such as the introduction of a $37\frac{1}{2}$ hour week and 18 month training courses for midwives, may tend to reduce the validity of year-to-year comparisons.)

III.14 There were considerable differences, however, between broad specialty groupings. The proportion of qualified staff in general nursing (ie acute and geriatric nursing) and maternity services actually increased between 1970 and 1977. By contrast, there was a sharp shift in mental handicap and mental illness fields in favour of unqualified staff. There is also a general shortage of staff in these fields, and this partly explains the increase in unqualified staff. The mental health field tends to be relatively unattractive to nurses, and the position has been worsened for the mental handicap sector by uncertainty over the Jay Report (still under consideration) which recommends that existing mental handicap nurses be replaced by staff with a new role providing social, rather than nursing, care in small group homes.

III.15 Community nursing staff are mainly registered or enrolled nurses. The proportion that nursing auxiliaries form of community nursing staff has risen in recent years but was still less than 5 per cent in 1977. In 1977, 509 district nurses (43 per cent of the total) did not hold the district nursing qualification. It is hoped that the introduction of mandatory training for district nurses will remedy this, but the present district nursing force may be depleted while training is carried out.

III.16 Taking into account the contribution of combined duty nurses, the present district nursing complement in most, but not all, health board areas exceeds the Department's minimum target ratio of 1 per 4,000 population. However, half the boards fail to meet the corresponding ratio of 1 : 4,600 for health visitors (which does not include any allowance for school nursing). Moreover, these minimum ratios do not allow for those areas where special health care is needed or where there is a highly developed scheme of attachment to general practice for which the Department's recommended ratios are 1 : 3,000 for health visitors and 1 : 2,500 for district nurses.

(iv) **Paramedical therapeutic manpower**

III.17 The paramedical therapeutic group (1977 whole-time equivalent in brackets) comprises speech therapists (214) and the professions supplementary to medicine viz: chiropodists (333), dietitians (104) orthoptists (44), radiographers (therapeutic) (74) and the remedial professions–occupational therapists (307), physiotherapists (822) and remedial gymnasts (28). Chiropodists and speech therapists are based mainly in the community, the others in hospitals. An associated group is made up of prosthetists and orthotists, but few are employed at present within the NHS.

III.18 There is no hard information on the overall need for paramedical therapeutic staff, but there is a general impression that there is at present a shortage of staff, particularly for the remedial professions and chiropodists. Although numbers of paramedical therapeutic staff have increased over the last 10 years, there have been problems with competition from social work authorities for occupational therapists and from private practice for chiropodists. As regards chiropodists, the NHS is unlikely ever to match the rewards of private practice (except for pension arrangements) so that the NHS will have to continue to rely on the services of private practitioners to a large extent. This costs more, in remuneration at least, than does direct employment of chiropodists.

III.19 If our recommendations that priority be given to the elderly, the mentally handicapped, the mentally ill and the physically handicapped are accepted, the demand for paramedical therapeutic manpower will increase. This demand would also be affected by the need to develop an effective community service which will arise from the proposed shift from hospital to community care. There are high wastage rates in both training and employment, which seem to call for investigation and action. As regards employment, there is scope, as noted in the General Manpower Survey in Chapter III(A)(i) above, for making more provision for women with domestic commitments, since most paramedical therapeutic staff are women.

III.20 Although the need for the services of paramedical therapists may be expected to increase, the financial resources available will determine how many can be employed. We note that the Royal Commission on the NHS has recommended an independent review of the machinery set up by the Professions Supplementary to Medicine Act 1960 and that it should include the training and manpower needs of these professions and speech therapists (paragraphs 15.7, 15.57). The Royal Commission also suggests that more use be made of ancillary help in chiropody (paragraph 8.31).

(v) **Clinical psychology manpower**

III.21 Our recommendations with regard to the elderly, the mentally handicapped, the mentally ill and the physically handicapped also have implications for clinical psychologists who are already in short supply. Although there is no shortage of applicants, training needs for this profession present serious funding problems which need examination.

(vi) Administrative and clerical manpower

III.22 There has been much concern in recent years about the rapid growth in administrative and clerical staff. As already recorded in the General Manpower Survey in paragraph III.3 above, administrative and clerical staff were one of the fastest growing groups over the period 1967–77, at 6.8 per cent per annum (compound).

III.23 So far as hospital-based staff are concerned, the growth of administrative and clerical staff must not be assumed to be synonymous with a growth in the number of administrators. The groups as defined in these statistics include staff, eg computer operators, who do not undertake administrative and clerical work, and functional managers, eg laundry managers. Moreover, of the 6,132 (whole-time equivalent) administrative and clerical staff based in hospitals at September 1977, 5,394 (88 per cent) were clerical, secretarial, typing and machine grades and included staff such as medical secretaries, ward clerks and medical records staff who provide direct support for clinical departments. Much of the growth in numbers, particularly after 1974, was due to commendable improvements in services, namely:

(a) expansion of operational services requiring an administrative input, eg better appointment and recall facilities for out-patient clinics;

(b) the use of administrative and clerical staff, eg medical records clerks, to relieve professional staff of non-professional duties, on the ground that highly skilled and expensive professional staff should not be required to devote time and energy to non-professional matters;

(c) the adoption of new technology, eg computerisation, and the introduction or expansion of specialist functions such as finance and personnel in order to provide adequate management for the reorganised NHS.

III.24 So far as non-hospital-based staff are concerned, the figures have been distorted by the absence of reliable figures before 1970 and by the transfer of staff from other authorities to the NHS on reorganisation in 1974.

III.25 If the staffing levels of health boards are compared by relating total administrative and clerical staff (whole-time equivalent) to revenue expenditure (on the basis that the need for such staff is related to the total volume of services provided and this is roughly measured by revenue expenditure), it is found that in 1977 the numbers of staff per £1 million total revenue expenditure (excluding family practitioner service expenditure) varied from 13.8 to 23.3. There are probably good explanations for some of these wide variations between boards which require further investigation. They could be due to differences in management style, the number of districts being administered and the geographical nature of the areas.

III.26 The most effective approach in seeking to contain costs of administrative and clerical staff is not to try to deal with the heterogeneous mass of such staff as one group, but to seek to control the numbers of those engaged in operational duties, eg medical records clerks, as part of the separate operations on which they are engaged, and for the rest to concentrate on general management costs. Following a report by a Working Party of Departmental and NHS Officers, set up by SHHD in 1976, the Secretary of State has decided that for the financial year 1979/80 each health board's expenditure on management and administration, expressed as a percentage of the board's total revenue expenditure for that year, should not exceed the percentage set out in the Department's NHS Circular No 1979(GEN)42, which also defines the items to be included in management and administrative costs.

(vii) Points deserving attention

III.27 The following points in connection with manpower seem to us to warrant particular attention:

(i) From our suggestions that priority be given to certain services and that within services certain objectives be set, there will arise the need to seek some redistribution of NHS staff between services to accord with these priorities and objectives. Steps must therefore be taken to facilitate such redistribution;

(ii) Solutions to the problems of geographical maldistribution of manpower which are apparent must be sought;

(iii) There is a need for better manpower planning within the Scottish Health Service; in particular, there is a need to find ways and means of reducing excessive wastage rates among certain categories of staff;

(iv) Using the Department's current minimum target ratios for district nurses and health visitors to population (see paragraph III.16 above), an increase in numbers of district nurses and health visitors will be necessary to enable these ratios to be met in all boards, and more community nurses will also be needed to meet the extra demands, eg the increasing numbers of over 75s, discussed in Chapter II. Meeting these requirements will only be possible if community nursing services are given a high priority;

(v)   More paramedical therapeutic staff and clinical psychologists will be required if our recommendations that priority be given to the elderly, the mentally handicapped, the mentally ill and the physically handicapped are to be achieved.

(B)   FINANCE

Introduction

III.28 This section briefly reviews past trends in NHS expenditure and its distribution between services and client groups. While finance is one of the main constraints on NHS growth, it is certainly not the only one; in particular, staff shortages will often be more important. Nevertheless plans for the future development of the Scottish Health Service must take account of the likely growth in financial resources. There is every indication that future expenditure growth rates will be relatively low. Some growth is required simply to meet the effects of demographic trends, particularly the need for more long-term care for the elderly, to implement new technological developments and to cover the net additional running costs of already committed building projects. The indications are that the capital monies likely to be available up to 1986 are already fully committed by schemes in the Major Building Programme and by the basic allocation for Health Boards' Ordinary Building Programmes; the latter can finance only small capital schemes. Revenue developments involving little or no capital expenditure will depend upon the future rate of growth. These points are taken up more fully in Chapter VI.

Total gross expenditure by sector

III.29 Table III.3 shows gross revenue and capital expenditure on the Scottish Health Service at constant prices for 1970/71–1976/77 by sector. Total expenditure grew at the relatively high rate of 2.7 per cent per annum (compound) over the whole period, but fell in 1976/77 due to a decrease in capital expenditure in all sectors, and in revenue expenditure in the hospital sector only. 1976/77 was the first year in which cash limits were applied to the bulk of NHS expenditure, the major exception being family practitioner services. Cash limits are based on the allocations made under the Public Expenditure Survey plus a fixed allowance to cover pay and price increases estimated to occur during the financial year. In 1976/77 price movements were greater than

Table III.3 NHS (Scotland) Expenditure§ Gross of FPS Charges by Category 1970/71–1976/77–At 1976 Survey Prices (£m)

Type of Expenditure	Category	70/71	71/72	72/73	73/74	74/75	75/76	76/77	% increase per annum compound 70/71–76/77
Current Expenditure (net)§	Hospital Services* Community Health Service	380.1	399.1	409.2	434.5	437.4	454.3	451.5	+2.9%
		26.6	29.3	30.4	33.6	35.1	35.4	36.8	+5.5%
	Family Practitioner Services†	113.8	114.1	123.0	123.4	125.3	134.9	138.3	+3.3%
	HB Administration‖	19.5	20.8	22.5	23.6	24.2	26.7	26.7	+5.4%
	Other‡	32.2	31.0	31.6	34.4	35.2	38.0	38.1	+2.8%
Capital Expenditure (net)	Hospital Services Community Health Services	44.8	46.7	58.1	52.6	47.3	42.3	35.3	−3.9%
		1.6	2.6	4.6	4.3	3.5	5.4	4.1	+17.5%
	Central Health Services¶	3.6	3.5	5.2	3.7	4.0	5.2	4.7	+4.3%
Total Current Expenditure§		552.7	573.5	594.2	625.9	633.0	662.6	664.7	+3.1%
Total Capital Expenditure (net)		50.0	52.8	67.9	60.6	54.8	52.9	44.1	−2.1%
Total Expenditure§		602.7	626.3	662.1	686.5	687.8	715.5	708.8	+2.7%

Sources: Scottish Office Finance Division; Scottish Health Statistics 1977, Table 10.1.

*Including costs of Health Board and Clinical Administration.
†Gross, excluding charges.
‡Expenditure on CSA, other central services eg research, training and central administration.
§Gross of charges listed under FPS.
¶Includes State Hospital.
‖Already included under Hospital Services.

allowed for in the cash limits, and boards had to reduce expenditure in real terms to compensate for this; and underspending occurred owing in part to the introduction of an arrangement enabling limited revenue funds to be carried over into the next financial year.

III.30 As regards the distribution of revenue expenditure by sector, the main change is the gradual decline of the proportion going on the hospital services since 1972/73. (See Table III.3). Nevertheless community health service revenue expenditure was still only $5\frac{1}{2}$ per cent of the total in 1976/77, compared with 68 per cent for hospital services. The hospital sector however includes the major element of the NHS commitment towards services for the elderly, the mentally handicapped and the mentally ill, all of which were given priority in 'The Way Ahead'. Family practitioner services have continued to take approximately one-fifth of all expenditure.

III.31 A similar change has occurred for capital expenditure, with the hospital sector's share falling from 90 per cent to 80 per cent between 1970/71 and 1976/77, while community health service expenditure has risen from 3 per cent to 10 per cent of the total (though this is an increased share of a reduced total).

Hospital services

III.32 Table III.4 shows the division of hospital running costs in 1976/77 between the long-term care services (chronic sick/geriatric, mental illness and mental handicap), acute services, and maternity services. It will be noted that in round figures 60 per cent of the total expenditure went on the acute and maternity services, and 40 per cent on the long-term care group.

Community health services

III.33 These services can be divided into five main groups: health centres and clinics; the care of mothers and young children; community nursing services; school health services; and general preventive services including, among other items, fluoridation, screening, health education, vaccination and immunisation. In 1976/77 health centres and clinics accounted for 15.9 per cent of running costs of community health services; care of mothers and young children for 5.0 per cent; community nursing services for 47.7 per cent; school health services for 19.8 per cent; and general preventive services and miscellaneous for 11.6 per cent.

Table III.4 Hospital Costs at actual prices by Broad Specialty Grouping 1976/77

Broad Specialty Grouping	Costs (£m)	% of Total Costs
Acute	201.95	51.8
Maternity	29.53	7.6
Chronic/Geriatric	61.17	15.7
Mental Illness	73.99	19.0
Mental Handicap	23.08	5.9
Total	389.73	100.0

Source: ISD, February 1979.
NHS Accounts 1976/1977

Note: The total cost shown comprises:

Total Hospital Running Expenses excluding theatre costs, diagnostic radiographers and rates and feu duties. [Statement C NHS Accounts 1976/77] and excluding non-salary administration costs [Statement B] plus Specialist Service Expenditure [Statement D] (References to statements are to NHS Accounts).

Family practitioner services

III.34 As Table III.5 shows, gross expenditure on the family practitioner services at constant prices grew by 21.5 per cent between 1970/71 and 1976/77, but the increase varied considerably between services. General medical services and general dental services grew by the relatively low amounts of 17 per cent and 13 per cent respectively while general ophthalmic services grew by 23 per cent and the general pharmaceutical service by 27 per cent. Expenditure on the family practitioner services is demand led in the sense that the level of services provided is by and large not subject to budgetary control. Therefore the differing growth rates for the various family practitioner services cannot be seen as embodying conscious decisions on priorities by the health authorities. However they can be regarded as giving some idea of trends in expenditure on these services.

III.35 Charges (ie income from patients) cover a large percentage of gross expenditure for the general dental and ophthalmic services (25 per cent and 37 per cent respectively in 1976/77) but cover only a small and declining share of gross expenditure in the general pharmaceutical service (4 per cent in 1976/77) though the July 1979 increase in charges will raise this share slightly from 1979/80 onwards.

Table III.5 Gross Expenditure on Family Practitioner Services 1970/71–1976/77 – £000s at Constant November 1976 Prices

Service	1970/71	1971/72	1972/73	1973/74	1974/75	1975/76	1976/77	Increase 1970/71–76/77
General Medical Services	34,073	34,590	35,269	35,819	37,100	39,063	39,785	16.8%
General Pharmaceutical Services	54,174	53,575	62,166	61,247	61,127	66,016	68,895	27.2%
General Dental Services	19,512	20,317	20,004	20,670	20,385	21,359	22,129	13.4%
General Ophthalmic Services	6,072	5,581	5,605	5,638	6,696	8,452	7,490	23.4%
All Family Practitioner Services	113,831	114,063	123,044	123,374	125,308	134,890	138,299	21.5%

Source: Scottish Office Finance Division.

54

Expenditure by programme

III.36 We asked that health boards be invited to provide information about (a) expenditure in the four financial years 1974/75–1977/78 on family practitioner services (FPS) and on each of seven health care programmes–child health, dental (ie excluding general dental services), elderly, maternity, medicine, mental and surgery–in hospital and in the community, and (b) activity data within these programmes (eg in-patient bed days, visits by health visitors). Most boards were able to provide information on expenditure, but some of those which responded were unable to provide reliable activity data for the earlier years except for hospital in-patients. Table III.6 summarises the expenditure at constant 1977/78 prices, grouping together for ease of presentation the acute service programmes, to which 'The Way Ahead' gave a low priority, and the long-term care services to which 'The Way Ahead' gave a high priority. (In Chapter VI we indicate our agreement with these broad priorities.)

III.37 We considered whether the trends in expenditure by programme might give some indication of the impact of 'The Way Ahead'. However, it was not published until April 1976 by which time the 1976/77 budgets had already been agreed, and while it could have altered expenditure patterns in 1977/78, this effect could well have been obscured by random year-to-year fluctuations. Instead we have examined trends in the distribution of expenditure over the whole period 1974/75–1977/78. As Table III.6 shows, expenditure on hospital services as a whole has grown twice as fast as community health expenditure as a whole, apparently contrary to the desired shift from hospital to community care. However this shift has occurred for the long-term care groups, for whom it is most important, with community health expenditure growing three times as fast as hospital expenditure. In absolute terms, however, most expenditure on these long-term services goes on hospital care. £12 million extra was spent on hospital services for this group in 1977/78 compared with 1974/75, and there was a growth of £2 million for community health services. We were disappointed to note that for hospital and community health services combined, expenditure on the acute service grew faster than expenditure on long-term care (and that the acute services used up over half of the total increase between 1974/75 and 1977/78), though the decrease in child health and maternity expenditure is in line with our priorities. Within the long-term group itself, there was increased expenditure on care of the elderly while expenditure on the mentally disordered remained more or less static. The only major change in hospital in-patient activity 1974/75–1977/78 was a sharp decline in discharges and occupied bed days in the child health programme.

Table III.6 Changes in Health Board Revenue Expenditure 1974/75–77/78. £m at constant 1977/78 prices

Type of Expenditure	Programme Group (individual programmes in group in brackets)	1974/75	1977/78	Change 1974/75–77/78 (£m)	Change 1974/75–77/78 (%)
	Acute (Medicine, surgery, dental)	197.5	215.6	+18.1	+9.2%
Hospital Expenditure	Long-term care (Care of elderly, mental)	146.3	158.2	+11.9	+8.1%
	Child	16.7	17.1	+0.4	+2.4%
	Maternity	31.3	31.5	+0.2	+0.8%
	All Programme Groups*	393.8	425.0	+31.2	+7.9%
	Acute (medicine, surgery, dental)	1.1	1.2	+0.1	+9.1%
Community Health Service Expenditure	Long-term care (care of elderly, mental)	7.9	9.9	+2.0	+25.3%
	Child	15.6	14.9	−0.7	−4.5%
	Maternity	5.2	4.6	−0.6	−11.5%
	All Programme Groups*	35.3	36.7	+1.2	+3.4%
	Acute (medicine, surgery, dental)	198.6	216.8	+18.2	+9.2%
Hospital and Community Expenditure	Long-term care (care of elderly, mental)	154.2	168.1	+13.9	+9.0%
	Child	32.3	32.0	−0.3	−0.9%
	Maternity	36.5	36.1	−0.4	−1.1%
	All Programme Groups*	429.1	461.7	+32.6	+7.6%
Family Practitioner Services		107.8	121.5	+13.7	+12.7%

Source: Working Party on Health Priorities from returns from health boards: Scottish Office Finance Division.

*Includes unallocable expenditure.

Table III.7 1978 Public Expenditure Survey Forecasts 1977/78–82/83

£m at 1978 Survey Prices

Category	Item	1977/78	1978/79	1979/80	1980/81	1981/82	1982/83	Average % growth (compound) pa 1978/79–82/83
Capital	Hospital and Community Health Services	39.3	46.5	45.0	46.0	48.8	54.1	3.9%
	Other health services*, †	4.7	4.9	5.4	5.1	6.0	6.5	7.3%
	Total capital	44.0	51.4	50.4	51.1	54.8	60.6	4.2%
Current	Hospital and Community Health Services	532.2	552.8	562.7	571.1	579.7	588.5	1.6%
	Family Practitioner Services	147.1	148.6	153.0	156.3	159.7	163.1	2.4%
	Other‡	42.9	45.9	46.6	47.1	47.6	48.1	1.2%
	Total Current	722.2	747.3	762.3	774.5	787.0	799.7	1.7%
	All Expenditure†	766.2	798.7	812.7	825.6	841.8	860.3	1.9%

Source: 1978 Public Expenditure White Paper Cmnd. 7439.

*Mainly central services eg CSA.

†Including expenditure incurred by Property Services Agency on services within the programme (£0.4 million in 1977/78, £0.3 million in 1978/79).

‡Includes health board administration, central health services, and miscellaneous items.

Future expenditure

III.38 The rate of expansion of the service in future will depend on Government decisions with regard to public expenditure. The expenditure plans of the last Government set out in the White Paper (Cmnd 7439) for the period up to 1982/83 were published in January 1979. The Scottish components of these figures are shown in Table III.7. The projected growth rate for all expenditure between 1977/78 (the financial year most nearly relating to the 1977 calendar year which forms the base year for this report), and 1982/83 is 2.4 per cent per annum (compound). However, this comparison gives a misleading impression of future national growth rates, as expenditure in 1977/78 was below trend. A more realistic comparison is between the estimates for 1978/79 and 1982/83, which gives a growth rate for all expenditure of only 1.9 per cent per annum (compound) compared with the 2.7 per cent growth rate between 1970/71 and 1976/77, and 3.5 per cent between 1970/71 and 1975/76. Revenue expenditure on hospital and community health services, which is directly controlled by health boards, is projected to grow at 1.6 per cent per annum (compound) nationally over the same period, while expenditure on the family practitioner services, which as noted above is demand-determined, is expected to increase by 2.4 per cent per annum (compound) between 1978/79 and 1982/83. Capital expenditure is projected to remain fairly steady between 1978/79 and 1980/81, but would then rise in the next two years to £54 million (converted into percentage growth rates, this would give a 4.2 per cent per annum (compound) increase for capital expenditure over the whole period 1978/79–1982/83 but given the year-to-year fluctuations this figure is not very meaningful). In planning the provision of buildings and equipment boards will, besides calculating the capital costs, have to assess carefully the revenue consequences which they will have to meet within their cash-limited revenue allocations.

III.39 These forecasts will in the normal way be reviewed in the Public Expenditure Surveys in the light of the Government's commitment (a) to maintain standards of patient care and (b) to reduce the rate of growth of public expenditure. The growth rates for individual health boards will also be affected by the implementation of SHARE. Table III.8 shows the adjustment which would have been required on the basis of the December 1978 target shares in order to bring health boards' allocations for 1978/79 into line with the targets. It will take many years to implement SHARE, and the targets will themselves change over time. However, on the basis of present information, Tayside (and Greater Glasgow if its population declines as expected) will experience growth rates significantly below the national rate, while Ayrshire and Arran and the Islands will benefit from significantly higher rates.

Table III.8 SHARE: Adjustments required to 1978/79 Estimated Final Allocations to achieve SHARE Targets

Health Board (1)	December 1978 Calculation Target Shares % (2)	1978–79 Estimated Final Allocation % of Scottish Total (3)	Adjustment required to achieve Parity (Column 2 less Column 3) (4)	Adjustment as % of 1978/79 Share of Estimated Final Allocation (Column 4 as a % of Column 3) (5)
Argyll and Clyde	7.31	7.21	+0.10	+1.4
Ayrshire and Arran	5.67	4.47	+1.20	+26.8
Borders	1.47	1.39	+0.08	+5.8
Dumfries and Galloway	2.60	2.54	+0.06	+2.4
Fife	4.79	4.54	+0.25	+5.5
Forth Valley	4.85	4.54	+0.31	+6.8
Grampian	8.90	8.60	+0.30	+3.5
Greater Glasgow	26.88	27.47	−0.59	−2.1
Highland	3.70	3.72	−0.02	−0.5
Lanarkshire	8.09	7.92	+0.17	+2.1
Lothian	15.65	16.40	−0.75	−4.5
Tayside	8.90	10.24	−1.34	−13.1
Islands	1.19	0.96	+0.23	+24.0
TOTAL	100.0	100.0	+2.70 −2.70	—

Sources: Scottish Office Finance Division, Planning Unit, SHHD.

IV Multiple Deprivation

Introduction

IV.1 Before considering priorities between programmes in Chapter VI we consider briefly, in this chapter and the next, two general priorities which cut across most services and client groups, ie multiple deprivation and prevention. Multiple deprivation has already been mentioned in individual programmes where special attention to multiply deprived areas seems to be required; and it was studied by a subcommittee of the Child Health Programme Planning Group. We now look at the health needs of multiply deprived households as a whole.

Priority for health needs associated with multiple deprivation

IV.2 Scotland has a disproportionate share of Great Britain's multiply deprived areas and, within these areas, the proportions of households with multiple deprivation are particularly high. Clydeside is the most severely deprived conurbation in Great Britain. We recognise that multiple deprivation has social and economic causes, eg poor housing conditions, which can be tackled only by local authorities and appropriate government departments. Nevertheless, there is evidence that multiple deprivation is associated with ill-health and, in turn, ill-health may lead to a deterioration in social circumstances. There is therefore a positive need to deal with the health problems associated with multiple deprivation and for health boards and their officers to give advice on the implications for health of the policies of other authorities for multiply deprived areas. 'The Way Ahead' commitment to giving priority to multiple deprivation should be reaffirmed. However it should be restated so as to define the role of health boards more clearly as follows: *'priority should be given by health boards, in association with other agencies, to dealing with the health problems associated with multiple deprivation.'*

Implementation of priority

IV.3 The most effective methods of implementing this priority will vary from locality to locality depending on the size and concentration of multiply deprived areas, the criteria used to define multiple deprivation, existing health facilities and the action taken locally by local authorities and government agencies towards relieving the social and economic factors giving rise to health problems. Each health board must decide as a matter of urgency its appropriate strategy in the light of local circumstances and in cooperation with local authorities and other government agencies.

IV.4 The following measures may form useful components of a programme for dealing with the health problems of the multiply deprived:

(a) The proposals for improving the coverage of ante-natal services and improvements in other maternity and neo-natal services discussed in the maternity services programme (paragraph II.41–47);

(b) Multiply deprived households can be encouraged to make more use of health services by providing facilities such as health centres in or near multiply deprived areas. At present travelling difficulties, particularly the cost and availability of public transport, may form a barrier to multiply deprived persons seeking health care. Where a multiply deprived area is too small to support permanent facilities of its own, it may be possible to provide services on a one or two days a week basis;

(c) Access to services may be improved by increasing their availability, eg by extending opening hours, in areas with a high concentration of multiply deprived households. Similarly, the uptake of services may be improved by increasing the attractiveness of health facilities;

(d) The most effective method of improving uptake may be the greater provision of domiciliary services, particularly the greater use of health visitors for preventive work and health education, and domiciliary family planning;

(e) Staff might be given special training for working with multiply deprived households, and also financial and other inducements (eg cars so that they need not use their own in areas with a high risk of vandalism) to apply for, and remain in, what is very demanding work;

(f) Consideration should be given to the introduction of programmes for selective screening of suitable groups in areas of multiple deprivation, and pilot schemes encouraged.

V Prevention

General

V.1 Many of the recommendations in our report stress the need for a change of emphasis towards prevention within the NHS. To achieve this change a major effort will be required. The maintenance of health has tended in the past to be equated with increasing the level of provision of health services but human biology, nutrition, lifestyle and the environment are at least equally important factors in achieving this aim. Lifestyle is probably the most important factor influencing health in Scotland today and we note that the White Paper 'Prevention and Health' published by the health departments in 1977 stressed the personal responsibility of the individual for maintaining his own health. Health education is the most important means of influencing behaviour.

V.2 There is evidence that health education has been most successful in Social Classes I and II which have responded to the need to modify behaviour more readily than other social classes. Likely explanations for this are that the level of education in these classes is higher and undesirable lifestyles are less acceptable in the environment in which they live and work. It is apparent to us that health education must be supplemented by other action if a major change in behaviour is to be effected in a large proportion of the population of Scotland. We now consider how such measures should be used in addition to health education in relation to smoking, alcohol abuse, and accidents.

Smoking

V.3 Cigarette smoking contributed to the 24,000 deaths from bronchitis, lung cancer and coronary heart disease (about 40 per cent of all deaths) which occurred in 1977. There is evidence that health education has had some success in persuading people to change their smoking habits, for example the switch from plain to filter cigarettes, the swing to low tar brands and the fact that fewer women smoke in pregnancy. On the other hand, there is evidence that young people are not being influenced by anti-smoking publicity. We think *fiscal measures would be the most potent way of discouraging smoking further*, for example not allowing the price of tobacco to fall relative to the retail price index or to real income. *Cigarette advertising should be more closely controlled. Further measures to restrict smoking in public to designated areas also might merit consideration.*

Alcohol abuse

V.4 Alcohol abuse is a growing problem in Scotland. As noted in paragraph II.67 admissions to mental hospitals for alcoholism have been growing rapidly, and alcohol often plays a role in crime and road accidents. We commend the Scottish Health Education Unit's campaign to increase public awareness of the nature of alcoholism and to encourage a belief in the possibility of recovery but, as for smoking, *fiscal measures to maintain the real cost of alcohol, and restrictions on advertising and sponsorship might prove more effective means of prevention.*

Ante-natal services

V.5 The uptake of ante-natal services is not as complete as could be desired (see Chapter II: Maternity and neo-natal services). Improvements in this field, and particularly in regard to neo-natal care, can lead to decreases in maternal mortality, perinatal and infant mortality, as well as ameliorating long-term handicap.

Road transport accidents

V.6 Road transport accidents are the greatest single cause of death among children and young adults, and are one of the three main causes of death in the 25–44 age group. They are also one of the main causes of physical handicap in the young age groups. We note that in the White Paper 'Prevention and Health' (paragraph 189), it is estimated that deaths and serious injuries to front seat occupants in car accidents could almost be halved if they wore their seat belts and *we strongly support the recommendation of the Royal Commission on the NHS in favour of the compulsory wearing of seat belts.* Other steps which would contribute to a reduction in the numbers and consequences of road accidents are measures to curb alcohol abuse (see paragraph

V.4) and publicity campaigns designed to increase public awareness of the seriousness of the road accident problem.

Fluoridation

V.7 We also wish to take this opportunity to reiterate our support in paragraph II.7 for the Royal Commission's recommendation that the Government should introduce legislation *to require water authorities to fluoridate water supplies at the request of health authorities.*

Role of health professionals

V.8 Apart from these measures, there is a need for all health professionals to make strenuous and continuing efforts to persuade patients to change their lifestyles and to accept the benefits of vaccination and immunisation. This presupposes that all health professionals are themselves convinced of the effectiveness of health education and it is not apparent to us that this is so. The dissemination of the results of scientifically controlled studies, which show both the practicability of changing the behaviour of patients and that such changes are in fact followed by improved health, might help to bring this about.

Role of health boards

V.9 It seems to us that health boards too must recognise they have an important role to play in prevention, especially in seeking to influence the many local authority services which control the environment. The environmental health and housing services of district authorities and the strategic planning, transport, water and leisure services of regional authorities have a profound effect on the health of the population they serve. Services provided to individuals by social work and education authorities also have an important influence on health. *Health boards must accept that it is their responsibility* to press upon local authorities the importance of these services in prevention.

Secondary prevention

V.10 Thus far we have discussed only primary prevention which is designed to prevent disease occurring. *We do not underrate however the importance of secondary prevention* which is concerned with the early detection and treatment of ill-health and usually takes the form of screening and/or periodic medical examinations of either selected groups of individuals at special risk or of unselected populations. For screening to be worthwhile there must be effective, acceptable tests for identification of the condition in its early stages; effective treatment and facilities to provide it; and a reasonable cost benefit return. Prevention also extends into clinical treatment designed to reduce disability and facilitate rehabilitation but this important aspect of prevention is not always recognised as such. There is a need, therefore, for every health professional to recognise that the tradition of equating the role of specific sections of the health professions such as community health doctors and health visitors with prevention is unduly restrictive; *all have an important role to play.*

VI Priorities

Introduction

VI.1 Having concluded that prevention and the health problems associated with multiple deprivation should have priority in the development of the Scottish Health Service as a whole, we turn to considering priorities between programmes. In this context, we are concerned only with service and client group programmes, because development of support services and the planning of manpower and other resources should be largely determined by the priority given to the health care programmes which make use of them. We wish to emphasise however that, whatever developments are planned either in services or in client group programmes, or in support services, the need to take account of, and to make proper provision for, the education and training of all types of staff, and for research, should be kept in mind at all times as an integral part of these developments.

VI.2 We should make it clear that the fact that a particular programme has not been awarded a high priority does not mean that it is not important but rather that, in comparison with other programmes, we do not consider it to merit expansion at this juncture. At the same time, there may well be objectives within such a programme that can and should be pursued. And a high priority for a programme does not imply that all its objectives should always take precedence over all objectives in a programme with a lower priority. In Chapter VII we consider which of the possible objectives within the various programmes could be achieved within the resources likely to be available.

Methodology

VI.3 To assist in its search for a scientific method of setting priorities, papers were presented to our Working Party on Health Priorities and a review of the literature was carried out for them. (In these activities the Scottish Institute for Operational Research played a large and useful role.) The common conclusion of all these was that no satisfactory scientific method of performing this task had yet been devised. Various methods for determining priorities, for example 'Criteria Models', had their advocates, but the Working Party concluded that, in the absence of wholly convincing research studies on the use of such methods to justify the adoption of any of them at this time, a pragmatic approach, in which value judgments would necessarily play a particularly large role, was best in present circumstances.

VI.4 We received reports and presentations on various aspects of the health service from Programme Planning Groups and National Consultative Committees, all of which provided helpful advice and information. All these reports, of course, set out what the respective Programme Planning Group or National Consultative Committee considered needed to be done within the programme or service with which each was concerned. Our task has been to review the whole health service and therefore to consider such reports in this wider context. In any event, value judgments necessarily play some part in all these reports, but such judgments by individual professional or other groups within the health service are not easy to harmonise. Moreover, the judgments of specialist groups within a profession may differ widely from the collective judgment of that profession, since those working in a specialty will see priorities which will not necessarily be shared by those working in another specialty. In addition, the preference of individuals within a profession for work within a particular branch of that profession is a limiting and often critical factor in giving effect to priorities. It should however be mentioned that the National Medical Consultative Committee in reporting upon the acute hospital services gave a most helpful analysis of the priorities which it considered should be accorded to the very varied problems within these services.

VI.5 Starting with the current list of priorities set out in 'The Way Ahead', we went on to consider for each service or client group whether, on the basis of national assessment, its relative priority should be changed in the light of such factors as expected demographic changes and discrepancies between the current level of services and what seemed the desirable level. The priorities suggested in 'The Way Ahead' were, apart from prevention and multiple deprivation:

(a) Promotion of health care in the community through the progressive improvement of primary care services and community health services;

(b) Lessening the growth rate of the acute sector of the hospital service;

(c) Continued improvements in hospital and community health services for the elderly, the mentally ill, the mentally handicapped and the physically handicapped.

VI.6 As noted in paragraph III.36, we obtained information on how the majority of health boards had spent revenue monies by programmes for the years 1974/75–1977/78. The short period following publication of 'The Way Ahead' in 1976 did not, of course, enable valid conclusions to be drawn on its effect on the programmes to which the Secretary of State wished priority to be given, but we noted that over the four year period there has been an increase in the share of expenditure going to care of the elderly. On the other hand the share of expenditure going to mental illness and mental handicap did not increase. Indeed, over the period a larger proportion of the growth monies in real terms went to the acute sector than to the combined programmes providing long-term care (mental illness, mental handicap and care of the elderly).

Primary health care

VI.7 We have taken this group to include general medical services, primary dental care (general and community dental services), general ophthalmic services, general pharmaceutical services and community nursing. A recurring theme in practically every programme considered in Chapter II, and in the various reports, is the need to care for more patients in the community. This is particularly important for patients requiring long-term care. Clearly, if adequate care is available in the community for these groups of patients so that they remain near to relatives and friends, it is better than admitting them needlessly to hospital. Even when hospitalisation is required it is desirable that they should be returned to the care of their family practitioner and community health services as soon as possible. This would reduce the demand on hospital services and enable the release of resources for use in other ways including at least some of the objectives listed in the acute services section of Chapter VII. This change from hospital to community care cannot take place overnight, and we cannot emphasise too strongly that particularly in the long-term care sector the critical factor will be the provision of appropriate local authority services, including residential accommodation, special housing, day centres and home helps. A positive integrated approach, in which health and local authorities coordinate their planning and share resources, is fundamental to the achieving of priorities to which the expansion of certain local authority services is essential (though we appreciate that local authorities are likely to be subject to even more severe financial constraints than health boards). Within the NHS the main burden will fall on the general medical services and community nursing services.

VI.8 The general medical services are on the whole reasonably adequate, though this is not true of every district and, as already noted in Chapter II, the role of general practitioners in prevention requires more emphasis. On the other hand, any expansion of community health care will put a heavy burden on the community nursing services, in which the numbers of nurses are already inadequate in some districts. Therefore, if the objectives for the community nursing services are to be achieved, there will have to be a very considerable expansion of staff numbers. This can only be done if, first, the finance is available to employ them, which would imply that expenditure on these services would grow much faster than expenditure on the health service as a whole; and, secondly, if the requisite numbers can be recruited and trained. On this second point, a considerable expansion has been achieved in the past, and it is to be hoped that a similar increase can be achieved in future. However, there may be local problems, and training facilities will be heavily in demand.

VI.9 As regards the other primary care services, there appears to be no major problem with the general ophthalmic service, or the provision of general pharmaceutical services, but we have already pointed to the need to seek to reduce the growth of expenditure on drugs. On the other hand, it is clear that the provision of primary dental care is less than adequate. However, as noted in Chapter II, dental services cannot be expanded rapidly because of limitations on the numbers of dental practitioners who can be trained by 1986. Action should be taken now to make better use of existing dental practitioners by increasing the numbers of dental ancillaries.

VI.10 In the longer term, the need for primary dental care would be considerably reduced by fluoridation of water supplies (or other supplementary means where fluoridation is not technically feasible). Fluoridation should therefore be vigorously pursued.

Acute hospital services

VI.11 Perhaps the most contentious principle in 'The Way Ahead' was to lessen the growth rate of the acute hospital sector. In recent years, however, there has been a considerable number of new medical and technological advances which cannot be denied to patients, even though a relatively small proportion of the population may be involved. The NMCC in their submissions to the Working Party indicated fields in which development is considered necessary. The NMCC in their report gave first priority to dealing with the problem of elderly patients occupying acute beds but who should properly be treated in long-stay hospitals or in the community. We recognise also that the growing numbers of over 75s will lead to an increase in the number of elderly patients requiring acute services, but this increase in numbers should be partially offset by the decrease in the 65–74 group and the shift within the rest of the adult population towards the younger, and healthier, age groups.

VI.12 There are several ways in which financial resources could be made available within the acute services to meet the cost of developments. The NMCC and NNMCC in their reports made reference to areas where they considered savings might be made. Beds at present occupied by patients no longer requiring treatment in acute hospitals could be released if alternative arrangements could be made for these patients. Above all, the same number of patients could be treated in fewer beds if length of stay and turnover interval were reduced. If such potential savings could be made it would prove possible to provide for some developments within the acute sector without increasing revenue expenditure, although some capital expenditure might be necessary.

Maternity services

VI.13 It now appears that the number of births will rise during the 1980s, though as yet it is impossible to be sure how large this increase will be. As already shown in Chapter II, if utilisation rates are sufficiently improved (and we believe they can be) the likely number of births can be accommodated within the existing number of obstetric beds. On the other hand, while some savings may be possible in favourable circumstances, these are unlikely to be sufficiently large to cover the costs of improving ante-natal services in order to reduce both perinatal mortality and handicap. Since such improvements are very important, the maternity services should be given the additional resources required to achieve them. Nevertheless the need for such extra resources should be kept under constant review, in the light of changes in utilisation rates and birth projections.

Child health

VI.14 Even with the rising birth rate, the child population will continue to fall for some years, particularly for older age groups, which would imply that the share of the available resources devoted to child health should be reduced. One counter-argument is that children are an investment for the future; another is that action to improve the health of children and prevent permanent handicap will reduce the burden on the NHS in future years. We accept the force of this latter argument, but we regard it as a case for selectively expanding preventive, screening and assessment services rather than all child health services. We consider that total resources in child health services should be increased to the extent that is called for to deal with the special problems of vulnerable families. In all other respects there should be a shift towards proven preventive and assessment services, and within the hospital services closure of in-patient units too small to meet the needs of children. This implies a concentration of in-patient facilities in the larger centres. To achieve such a concentration it would first be essential to make out-patient facilities more widely available. It should also be recognised that many of the objectives for the child health services have implications for other services, such as the community nursing services, which we have taken into account in formulating objectives for these services.

Elderly

VI.15 The impact of changes in the elderly population on the primary health care and acute hospital services has already been fully discussed. The large growth expected in the number of over 75s will put increasingly great pressure on resources for long-term care, both in the community (in the provision of which the cooperation of local authorities will be essential) and in geriatric hospitals and day hospitals. Priority must be given to meeting the demands arising from these demographic pressures, as well as from the need to improve existing services.

Elderly with mental disability

VI.16 Demographic changes will also result in an increase in the numbers of the elderly with mental disability, and extra provision will have to be made towards meeting this increase as well as existing unmet needs. We note that the Major Building Programme makes provision for additional beds and some existing beds are being replaced but the 1986 total would still fall substantially short of what the Programme Planning Group recommends (see paragraph II.62). Besides, some upgrading of present accommodation and expansion of services will be required. We indicate in Chapter VII how a start could be made towards meeting these deficiencies, and for the above reasons we accord top priority to meeting the needs of the elderly with mental disability.

Mentally handicapped

VI.17 While the prevalence of severe/moderate handicap appears to be increasing because patients are living longer, demographic changes will have little overall effect on demands for services for the mentally handicapped. There is however a need to reduce the dependence on hospital provision, and at the same time to replace or upgrade some existing hospitals. These developments will require additional resources, particularly capital, and these objectives can only be achieved if priority is given to the mentally handicapped. As there is a shortage of staff in this field, further incentives may be required to attract more recruits.

Mentally ill

VI.18 Services for adult mental illness have had a low priority in the past and there is considerable scope for improvement. A community-based service in which social work and voluntary services have an important role, allied to a modern hospital-based service, is essential, as are improvements in mental health services for children and adolescents. All of these point to mental illness meriting priority. Again, more staff will have to be induced to enter this field.

Physically handicapped

VI.19 Although much of the needs of the physically handicapped is met within community-based services (including those provided by voluntary agencies), there is a need to make more progress in the development of rehabilitation programmes for the physically handicapped. Continuing attention must be paid to placing the young chronic sick in appropriate accommodation and this may require new building or upgrading of existing hospital buildings. The physically handicapped programme should be given priority so that progress towards achieving these objectives can be made.

Summary

VI.20 We set out below a list of programmes by priority category, including prevention and multiple deprivation (see Chapters IV and V). Programmes within a given category are not set out in any specific order but, in general, health boards should give priority to Category A programmes over other categories and should plan for the implementation of priorities in Category C programmes according to their ability to make savings in the fields covered by these programmes. The assumption would be that revenue expenditure on Category A programmes would grow faster than all health service revenue expenditure; Category B programmes would grow but at a lower rate than Category A programmes; and expenditure on Category C programmes would remain almost static in real terms or actually decline (and expenditure on any developments within a Category C programme must be met from savings).

VI.21 It will be noted that in allocating programmes to priority categories, as set out below, we have included in Category A prevention, services for the multiply deprived and community nursing services. Prevention and multiple deprivation are different in kind from other programmes, since they are concerned with the way in which the health services as a whole are provided, and therefore help to determine priorities within all individual client groups and service programmes, including those placed in Categories B and C. On the other hand, objectives for the community nursing services will be affected by the objectives adopted for client group programmes. In addition, as community nurses play an important role in prevention and services for the multiply deprived, the high priority given to them in itself implies a high priority for community nursing services. Finally, we support 'The Way Ahead' in giving priority to continuing promotion of health care in the community; this will also increase the need for community nurses.

Category A: Prevention
Services for the multiply deprived
Community nursing services
Care of the elderly
Elderly with mental disability
Mentally ill
Mentally handicapped
Physically handicapped

Category B: Primary dental services (general dental services[1] and community dental services)
Maternity services
General medical services[1]
General ophthalmic services[1]

Category C: Child health
Acute hospital services
General pharmaceutical services[1]

---

[1]These family practitioner services are, of course, different from the others in that expenditure on them is generally not subject to control by health boards.

VII Programme Objectives

Introduction

VII.1 We now use the broad priorities established in Chapter VI, and information on the likely level of future resources, to examine the list of potential programme objectives, ie the underlined statements in Chapter II, and place them within priority categories. (For this purpose we distinguish between potential objectives involving substantial capital expenditure, chiefly those concerned with the provision of new and replacement beds, and those involving mainly revenue expenditure). We should make it clear that, in doing so, we are aware that our assumptions about growth rates are very vulnerable to factors such as inflation, which if present trends continue will be substantial. The likelihood that costs to be contained within cash limits on expenditure will be subject to unpredictable change could alter matters significantly. We should also stress that we are considering the national picture; health boards will properly have the major part to play in determining how expenditure is to be incurred in their respective areas. Nevertheless we think it is useful to examine the priorities and objectives we propose in the light of the resources that may be available. *Collaboration in planning and in the sharing of resources between health boards and local authority services is crucial to the success or failure of attempts to achieve the proposed objectives.* Failing close collaboration *at every level,* results will continue to fall far short of what is attainable given the same overall commitment in terms of finance and manpower. We welcome the inception of support financing in Scotland as a useful, if still modest, stimulus to an integrated approach on the part of health boards and local authorities.

Objectives involving major capital expenditure

Financial background

VII.2 In relation to health boards, the Capital Building Programme consists of two main elements. The Major Building Programme comprises schemes whose priority has been determined by the Secretary of State after consultation with health authorities. Schemes in the Major Building Programme have first charge upon available capital resources. The second main element is the Ordinary Building Programme, within which priorities are determined by the boards themselves, financed by an annual allocation made in proportion to crude population numbers. Any surplus funds (which arise mainly from planned expenditure on the Major Building Programme not being incurred because of site and other difficulties (ie 'slippage')) are distributed to boards as additions to their Ordinary Programme allocation according to need, or the ability to spend in a particular financial year. Since reorganisation the surplus funds distributed in this way have been very substantial, but from now to the end of the decade little or no extra money is likely to be available because of the over-commitment to the Major Building Programme discussed below in paragraph VII.4.

VII.3 We do not believe that crude population figures give an adequate measure of the needs which health boards have to meet under their Ordinary Building Programme, and *recommend that the formula for allocating money for the Ordinary Programme be reviewed.*

Major Building Programme

VII.4 The initial difficulties after NHS reorganisation in getting the Major Building Programme under way are slowly being overcome, and there has been a build up of committed projects. We learned that expenditure on these projects in the Major Building Programme alone seems likely to exceed the capital expenditure forecasts over the period to 1982/83 (the last year for which a forecast is available), the greatest excess occurring in 1981/82. This apparent excess of expenditure over the money available might lead to some committed projects having to be delayed but in practice the excess may be compensated for by slippage. While it may be possible to introduce extra projects into the programme after 1982/83 in order to bring it more closely in line with the priorities and objectives recommended in this report, these could hardly start for some years and would not become operational until late into the decade. Fortunately, since the guidelines set out in 'The Way Ahead' were taken into account in the last major revision of the Building Programme, completed in 1977, the majority of recently committed projects are already related to priority programmes. The new hospital beds being provided under the present Building Programme by the mid 1980s are mainly geriatric beds, together with a number of psychogeriatric and mental handicap beds. Provision is also made for a number of replacement beds in the mental handicap, psychiatric, geriatric and psychogeriatric fields, and this should produce some improvements in the quality of the existing stock: some provision is also made for day hospitals.

Ordinary Building Programme

VII.5 Little information is available centrally on projects included in the Ordinary Building Programme (except for health centres which are relevant to our primary health care objectives and on which information is held centrally) but this is not crucial since much of it is necessarily devoted to projects not directly relevant to the objectives discussed in this report. Moreover the over-commitment of the Major Building Programme in the next few years means that boards will no longer receive the additional allocations to their Ordinary Programme they have been receiving in the past few years due to underspending in the Major Programme.

Future planning

VII.6 In drawing up new guidelines for the period to 1986, we were restricted by our knowledge that objectives requiring substantial capital expenditure could not be implemented quickly. We think that the next planning round must look far enough ahead to allow for the planning, construction and commissioning of building projects to be carried out within the period covered by the guidelines. *We therefore recommend that national guidelines should be promulgated every five years to cover the subsequent 10 year period.*

Revision of Building Programmes

VII.7 If the next national guidelines are not issued for another five years, they will be too late to affect the Major Building Programme for the mid to late 1980s. To avoid this possibility we *strongly recommend that the Department begin a review of the Major Building Programme in conjunction with health boards as soon as the Secretary of State announces his guidelines in 1980.* This review should be based on our objectives involving substantial capital expenditure which are listed by programme in paragraph VII.8. It is possible that certain of these objectives, for example the provision of day hospitals, could be achieved by some health boards within their Ordinary Building Programme, even although the money available is less than in previous years. We therefore *recommend that each health board should combine a review of its Ordinary*

Building Programme with its contribution to the national review of the Major Building Programme. Such a combined review would also present an opportunity for the boards and the Department to consider whether, in view of the objectives involving building included in our list, more of the available resources should be allocated to the Ordinary Building Programme particularly after 1982/83. *We recommend that the review of the Ordinary and Major Building Programmes should include consideration of whether the division of the total capital allocation between the two programmes needs to be changed.*

List of objectives and the need for capital expenditure

VII.8 Our list of recommendations for objectives and the consequent need for capital expenditure is set out by programme below:

CATEGORY A

Prevention–minimal capital expenditure.

Services for the multiply deprived

Provide health centres or other health service facilities in or near multiply deprived areas (sometimes what will be required is re-siting of facilities rather than extra provision).

Community nursing services–no capital expenditure.

Care of the Elderly

(1) Provide 40 geriatric hospital beds per 1,000 population over age 75;
(2) Increase geriatric day hospital provision to 2.0 places per 1,000 population over age 65.

Elderly with mental disability

(1) Provide long-stay hospital beds for elderly with mental disability. (The Mental Disorder Programme Planning Group has estimated that 10 places per 1,000 population over age 65 will be required.)

(2) Provide additional psychogeriatric day hospital places. (The Mental Disorder Programme Planning Group has estimated 2.5 places per 1,000 population over age 65 will be required.)

Mentally ill

Continuation of the process of upgrading standards of accommodation and care in mental illness hospitals.

Mental handicap

(1) Continue upgrading of existing hospital accommodation;

(2) Geographical redistribution of beds aimed at providing services locally and thus reducing the size of very large hospitals.

Physically handicapped

Provide more hospital accommodation suited to the young chronic sick.

CATEGORY B

Maternity services – minimal capital expenditure.

Primary dental care – minimal capital expenditure.

CATEGORY C

Child health

(1) Extend out-patient facilities to peripheral hospitals and health centres, and make further provision for day patient facilities;

(2) Subject to achievement of (1), rationalise paediatric hospital in-patient services, closing units which are too small to meet the needs of children and maintain the medical and nursing skills of staff.

Acute hospital services

(1) Rationalise accident and emergency services;

(2) Develop oncology services (proposals involving major capital expenditure only, eg provision of 150 beds);

(3) Improve orthopaedic services and expand joint replacement surgery;

(4) Develop pacemaker services.

VII.9 It will be noted that the programmes have been arranged by the priority categories set out in paragraph VI.21. We would expect the money for capital developments for Category C services to be found from revenue savings achieved within these services. Programme objectives in Category A would in general receive the highest priority. We reviewed the numerous objectives within this category in the light of (a) the shortfall of provision below these objectives which would still exist in 1986 even if all the committed projects in the Major Building Programme expected to be in operation by that date opened on time, and (b) the general considerations set out in Chapter VI. We concluded that priority should go first to the elderly with mental disability, second to the mentally ill, mentally handicapped and the elderly, and third to remaining programmes in Category A with objectives involving building, ie services for the multiply deprived and the physically handicapped.

General considerations

VII.10 We would like to make two general points concerning the building programmes. First, wherever this can be done satisfactorily extra beds required for a particular service should be provided by converting existing beds, formerly used for services which under our proposals would require fewer beds, rather than by constructing new buildings. Second, flexible and efficient use should be made of existing beds by reducing rigid allocations between different specialties.

Hospital and community health service objectives not involving major capital expenditure

VII.11 We then examined the objectives for the hospital and community health services which could be implemented by the mid-eighties, because they involved either no capital expenditure, or only small amounts. We must reiterate the point made in paragraph VII.6 that our choice of objectives has been restricted by our knowledge that any objectives which would involve major capital building for the period up to 1986 could not be implemented by then. There were objectives, for example more hospital provision for the elderly with mental disability, which we would rather have seen achieved by 1986 than some of those recommended in this section, but we had to accept that there was little likelihood of their being implemented by that date.

VII.12 We were of the opinion that we should not include any potential objectives in our final list of recommendations without assessing both their costs, and the revenue which might be available on varying growth assumptions. To begin with we attempted to calculate the costs of potential objectives. It was in this area that we found the greatest difficulty. Only very approximate estimates of the costs of various proposals were possible and in very few cases could any judgment be made of the benefits likely to ensue from these outlays. We accept that the quantification of benefits is extremely difficult and although there is usually some information available, nevertheless the element of judgment in assessing possible benefits remains greater than we would wish.

VII.13 We estimated the financial resources available as follows:

(a) The extra revenue likely to be available in 1986/87 over the current financial year 1979/80 was calculated. Figures were available from the 1978 Public Expenditure Survey, but only up to 1982/83. Since the position after that date is unknown, three different forecasts were produced for hospital and community health service revenue, ie (1) a central forecast, continuing the 1978/79–1982/83 growth rate of about $1\frac{1}{2}$ per cent up till 1986/87; (2) a high forecast on the same basis but using a 3 per cent growth rate, and (3) a low forecast assuming nil growth after 1982/83.

(b) The above forecasts were adjusted to take account of (1) the revenue consequences of committed major building projects allowing for probable slippage, and delays in bringing buildings fully into operation; (2) the revenue expenditure resulting from the decision to implement the Cardiac Surgery Programme Planning Group report; and (3) an allowance to cover such items as new statutory obligations, and new developments in medical technology and changing medical practice.

(i) **Nil growth assumption**

VII.14 Under the nil growth assumption, bearing in mind that there would be $1\frac{1}{2}$ per cent growth until 1982/83, it would be possible up to that date to

80

provide across the country as a whole for the revenue consequences of major capital projects, for the items mentioned in VII.13(b), and perhaps for some minor developments. However, after that period and until 1986/87 it would not be possible to provide even for these revenue consequences except by making substantial savings. We identified the following examples of areas where possible savings could be made:

Acute services

(1) Reduce the ratio of acute beds to population;

(2) Introduce hospital formularies for drugs;

(3) Introduce more discriminating use of existing radiological and laboratory investigations.

Child health

Close hospital in-patient units too small to meet the needs of children and maintain the medical and nursing skills of staff.

Maternity services

(1) Reduce the length of post-natal stays in the maternity services;

(2) Close under-used maternity beds.

However, most of the potential savings in the maternity services will possibly be swallowed up if the projected increase in births occurs and, in unfavourable circumstances (see paragraph II.46 and Table II.2), there could be a net increase in maternity services expenditure.

(ii)   1.5 per cent growth assumption

VII.15 All the net growth money available under this option should be allocated to services placed in Categories A and B in Chapter VI. From our calculations it seems probable that there would be sufficient finance available to achieve all the objectives in these categories not requiring capital expenditure, though their achievement may be hindered by staffing and other constraints. We realise however that the financial position of boards will vary because of the effects of SHARE and the need to budget for the revenue consequences of committed projects. We decided therefore to divide our objectives into lists 1 and 2 in the belief that all boards will have sufficient finance to accomplish those in list 1, subject to staff constraints, and that most boards will be able to include all or some in list 2. Within these lists we do not put objectives in any particular order of priority. We went on to add a further list 3 (self-financing) which are developments we regard as highly desirable but which should be financed (including capital expenditure required) by the savings already mentioned in paragraph VII.14. Our reason for adding this list is our acceptance that in a period of slow growth money saved in the acute or child health services should be used in the first instance to finance priority developments in that service.

LIST 1

(1) Put more emphasis on the preventive measures listed in Chapter V, particularly:

    (a) health education, especially programmes aimed at modifying unhealthy behaviour, and also dental health education;

    (b) water fluoridation.

(2) Improve services to multiply deprived households (see Chapter IV).

(3) Maintain and expand community nursing services to:

    (a) meet the needs of the increasing numbers of over 75s in the population;

    (b) meet the increased emphasis on prevention and health education;

    (c) meet the shift from hospital to community care, including the expansion of community services for the mentally ill and the mentally handicapped.

(4) Improve uptake of ante-natal services by encouraging earlier ante-natal attendances by all practical means. (This would be in addition to such improvements in areas of multiple deprivation under item 2 above.)

(5) Implement the recommendations of the Joint Working Party on Standards of Perinatal Care relating to organisation and professional practice, and make similar improvements in neo-natal services, particularly special or intensive care. As part of these improvements maternal serum alphafetoprotein screening should be made available routinely to all expectant mothers in Scotland.

LIST 2

(1) Introduce 'augmented home care' subject to satisfactory outcome of current evaluation – as part of policy of keeping elderly in the community.

(2) Expand the community-based services for mental illness by means of a joint planning approach by the health service and local authorities in liaison with voluntary agencies.

(3) Extend home visiting (ante- and post-natal) by midwives and health visitors to mothers at risk.

(4) Expand the child and adolescent psychiatry services.

(5) Prepare an overall plan to coordinate the growth and development of services for the physically handicapped, with the general aim of improving community services to enable the physically handicapped to live at home wherever possible.

(6) Ensure young chronic sick in hospital are placed in suitable accommodation.

(7) Promote a more even geographical distribution of dentists.

(8) Improve the efficiency of the dental care team by more use of dental ancillaries.

(9) Increase supply of skilled shoemakers producing orthopaedic footwear.

In this paragraph objectives (7) and (8) above refer to community dental services, but they depend in part upon what happens within the general dental services (see paragraph VII.17 below).

LIST 3 – SELF FINANCING

Child health

Introduce pilot projects to evaluate improvements in health surveillance of all children, comprehensive developmental screening of pre-school children and assessment of handicapped children recommended by Child Health Programme Planning Group (and, if proven, introduce as finance allows). This will also create a need for additional community nurses.

Acute services

(1) Improve orthopaedic services and expand joint replacement surgery.

(2) Develop oncology services.

(3) Improve services for sexually transmitted diseases.

(4) Develop urological services with rationalisation of renal transplant surgical services.

(5) Develop pacemaker services.

(6) Rationalise accident and emergency services.

(iii) 3 per cent growth rate

VII.16 We considered whether we should make further recommendations for new developments to be introduced if the 3 per cent growth rate was achieved. We thought it would be more useful to transform the extra revenue into additional capital expenditure. This would allow more rapid progress to be made towards meeting the shortfall of actual provision (even allowing for committed projects in the building programme) below that required to achieve the objectives involving substantial capital expenditure set out in paragraph VII.8. *We recommend that if a 3 per cent growth rate becomes possible, the difference between the $1\frac{1}{2}$ per cent and the 3 per cent growth rate should be used to increase capital expenditure, and make allowance for the revenue consequences of that increase.*

Family practitioner services

VII.17 We have omitted any consideration of family practitioner services in this context, since they are demand led and the method of financing them is different. Nevertheless, there are savings to be made in the use of drugs in general pharmaceutical services which we hope could be used to offset additional expenditure on the undernoted developments within the family practitioner services:

General medical services

(1) Greater emphasis should be placed on preventive medicine.

(2) The concept of the primary care team (which includes social work involvement) and the trend towards practitioners working in groups from shared premises should continue to be actively supported.

General dental services

(1) Promote a more even geographical distribution of dentists.
(2) Improve the efficiency of the dental care team by encouraging more use of dental ancillaries within the general dental services.

(The extent to which these objectives are implemented within the general dental services will affect the need to implement objectives (7) and (8) in list 2 in paragraph VII.15 above within the community dental services.)

General ophthalmic services

Improve services to the housebound, elderly and handicapped, both in the community and in long-stay accommodation.

General practice pharmaceutical services

(1) Continue to monitor the availability and distribution of general practice pharmaceutical services at local level.
(2) Ensure maximum economy in the drug bill.

Appendix 1

An estimate of possible saving by reducing D G H bed complement to that recommended in 'The Way Ahead'

1. This paper estimates the possible saving in cost that would result from reducing the bed complement in DGH specialties to the level of 2.5 beds per 1,000 population as recommended in 'The Way Ahead', a reduction of approximately 4,000 beds. It is assumed that the current level of patient discharges will be maintained. Table 1 below shows the present and proposed situations:

Table 1

	(a) 1978 situation	(b) Proposed situation
Bed complement in DGH specialties	16,954	12,949
Bed complement per 1,000 population	3.3	2.5
Discharges (including deaths and transfers)	470,821	470,821
Staffed beds	16,353	12,500
Occupied beds	12,148	10,000
Occupancy ratio	74%	80%
Throughput	29	38
Turnover interval	3.3	1.9
Mean stay	9.4	7.8

2. To maintain the current level of discharges with fewer beds, the throughput must increase. This can only be achieved by reducing the length of stay of the patients and/or increasing the occupancy of the staffed beds. Column (b) shows that to achieve the reduced bed complement the occupancy ratio has been assumed to increase from 74 per cent to 80 per cent; mean stay has been assumed to fall from 9.4 to 7.8 days and the turnover interval from 3.3 to 1.9 days. Given these changes, throughput increases from 29 to 38 cases per bed per annum.

3. The resultant changes in costs have been considered in relation to four components of hospital costs:

(1) Medical staff–it is assumed that these remain the same to cope with the same number of discharges.

(2) Nursing staff–these will fall because of the lower number of beds but not on a pro-rata basis (see paragraph 7 below).

(3) Hotel and other costs–the savings will vary according to the fixed or variable nature of the cost (see paragraph 8 below).

(4) Other treatment costs (eg pharmacy, theatre)–these are assumed not to change as they vary directly with the number of patients treated.

4. Table 2 below shows the costs at 1977/78 prices estimated for these components at present and given the proposed reduction in number of beds:

Table 2

	£ Present	£ Proposed
1. Medical staff total	16.8m	16.8m
per staffed bed	1,026	1,244
2. Nursing staff total	45.35m	41.35m
per staffed bed	2,773	3,308
3. Hotel and other costs total	70.5m	62.4m
per staffed bed	4,312	4,992
4. Other treatment costs total	47.5m	47.5m
per staffed bed	2,906	3,802
Estimated DGH bed cost total	180.15m	168.05m
per staffed bed	11,016	13,444

Source: SHSC year ended March 1978.

NB. This table estimates only the DGH costs. The teaching element of acute bed provision has been assumed to remain constant.

5. The possible savings are then as follows:

Nurses	£4.0m
Hotel costs	£8.1m
Total savings	£12.1m

Thus, although the initial reduction of 4,000 in the bed complement implies saving 25 per cent of beds, this may result in a saving of only 18 per cent in occupied beds and because of increased patient cost per bed, an overall cost saving of only 6.7 per cent of current cost.

6. The average numbers of available staffed beds in the DGH specialties in the year ended 30 September 1978 are:

DGH specialty

General surgery	3,952
Orthopaedic surgery	2,823
ENT surgery	739
Ophthalmology	519
Urology	441
Gynaecology	1,360
Dental surgery	62
Paediatric surgery	332
Paediatric medicine	665
General medicine	4,473
Respiratory medicine	654
Dermatology	333
Total DGH	16,353

Source: Information Services Division (ISD)(S)(1).

7. Hospital cost component 2 – nursing staff

If nurse ratios were to remain constant (at 1.39 per occupied bed) then the reduction in beds identified in Table 1 would imply a considerable fall in the number of nurses; if the number of nurses remained constant on the other hand the ratio would rise to 1.69 per occupied bed. The increased throughput and reduced mean stay mean that average patient dependency will increase and the nursing care required will become more intensive. Allowance must also be made for an increase in nursing duties outside the wards, for example in operating theatres which would need to work more intensively. For these reasons a 'middle-line' assumption is used: namely that the increase in nurses required to cope with the more intensive workload would offset half of the decrease in nursing staff requirements resulting from the reduction in occupied beds. In terms of the nurse ratio this indicates a ratio of 1.54 per occupied bed compared with the 1978 figure of 1.39, and with the ratio of 1.69 which would result if there was no reduction in nursing staff. Applied to the reduced bed numbers the 1.54 ratio gives a net saving of 1,500 nurses and a resulting money saving of approximately £4.0 million. (Estimated average cost per nurse per year equals £2,680 at 1977/78 prices.)

8. Hospital cost component 3 – hotel and other costs

Five costing groups were identified and an appropriate scaling factor applied to the present costs of each of them as follows:

Costing Group	Scaling Factor
(i) staff catering, administration and residences	the present cost per staffed bed is increased by the change in staffing ratios, ie 1.1
(ii) patient catering	the total cost is adjusted by the ratio of the proposed to present number of occupied beds, ie 0.8
(iii) other patient services (eg laundry, admin and records)	the total cost is expected to remain constant since this cost varies with the number of discharges
(iv) cleaning, domestic	the cost per staffed bed is assumed to remain the same since wards are unlikely to be cleaned more frequently
(v) fabric running and heating costs (eg steam production, engineering)	the probable change in costs will depend largely on the policy adopted to achieve the reduction in beds. Where hospitals are closed these running costs disappear whilst where wards are closed and not redeployed the running cost per staffed bed will increase. It is assumed here that overall there may be some increased cost per bed and for simplicity the factor used in (i) was used, ie 1.1.

Appendix 2

Support Services

(i) Scientific Services

1. *Radiodiagnostic services* are provided mainly at acute hospitals, but also at certain clinics and health centres. General practitioners in many parts of Scotland have 'open access' to X-ray facilities in hospitals and clinics. In addition to services provided in NHS buildings, four mass miniature radiography (MMR) units are available to serve the whole country as needed.

2. New attendances at diagnostic radiology departments annually are rather more than 1 million, of which 0.175 million are by hospital in-patients. Total attendances are about 2 million, of which 0.5 million are by in-patients. Attendances at MMR units have fallen steadily over the years and in 1977 were 0.159 million, ie about half of the number of attendances in 1965, reflecting the reduction in incidence and prevalence of tuberculosis. The units are now used for X-rays of groups considered to be most at risk of contracting tuberculosis.

3. The cost of individual items of X-ray equipment varies from about £1,000 for relatively simple apparatus to up to £0.5 million for whole-body scanners, and maintenance and replacement of equipment is a substantial commitment.

4. *Ultrasonography* has developed rapidly in the last 10 years or so, and one or more machines are in use in all health board areas except the Northern Isles. Statistics of usage are not collected centrally, but there are indications that usage of ultrasound is continuing to increase through expansion into fields other than obstetrics, in which it was first introduced, without a corresponding fall in usage of diagnostic X-ray facilities.

5. The report on 'Future Development of Ultrasound in Scotland' produced jointly by the National Medical Consultative Committee (Specialty Sub-committee for Radiology) and the National Consultative Committee of

Scientists in Professions Allied to Medicine (Medical Physics and Bio-engineering Subcommittee) recommended that ultrasound machines be located mainly in or adjacent to radiodiagnostic departments, even although ultrasound will not be a procedure to be used exclusively by radiologists.

6. The principal function of *medical laboratory services* is to assist clinicians (hospital doctors and to an increasing extent general practitioners) in diagnosis and the control and monitoring of therapy. Demand is therefore an outcome of the range of tests offered (which should reflect the needs of clinicians) and the frequency with which each is requested by clinicians. Another important function is the provision of support for epidemiological services. The principal disciplines are haematology, clinical chemistry, histopathology and microbiology (of which virology is a sub-group); immunology is a developing specialty, currently provided from laboratories in different disciplines.

7. Services are provided on an area basis, normally by the health board, but in areas with a medical school, services may be provided by a joint University/NHS laboratory or on an agency basis by the University. Certain laboratories providing local services also act as a national or regional reference laboratory.

8. Although measurement of laboratory work is not easy, there is evidence that the workload in clinical chemistry, haematology and microbiology has grown rapidly in recent years, but the availability of automated equipment, particularly in clinical chemistry and haematology, and discrimination in the use of laboratory services, has enabled laboratories to cope with the increased workload without a comparable increase in staff. New medical practices and techniques making use of laboratory investigations in acute, preventive and community health services may increase workload demands and create pressures for greater manpower and equipment resources.

9. Implementation of the new 'Code of Practice for the Prevention of Infection in Clinical Laboratories', for which the final target date is March 1982, may create some financial problems.

10. The radiodiagnostic, ultrasonography and laboratory services must respond to the needs of the clinical services, but there is scope for savings *by:*
(a) Eliminating unnecessary examinations. Local monitoring committees of clinicians can be of help here. Although many examinations may stem from a fear of litigation, the adoption of codes of practice might offer

some defence to clinicians and also assist in reducing the number of examinations.

(b) Eliminating outmoded techniques once new techniques have been proved. *Regular critical review to assess the value of individual investigations to patient management should be undertaken.*

(c) Introducing machinery at national level to advise on the purchase of sophisticated and expensive equipment.

(d) Good liaison between clinicians and laboratory consultants, especially where facilities are centralised.

The savings effected by these measures should in the main be used to finance new developments within the radiodiagnostic and laboratory services, although there would be merit in diverting a proportion of any monies saved into the clinical areas as an incentive for change in their demands on these services.

11. *The Scottish National Blood Transfusion Service* (SNBTS) is one of the Divisions of the Common Services Agency covering the whole of Scotland through five regional centres. In addition there is a Protein Fractionation Centre (PFC) which processes plasma provided by the regional centres.

12. The responsibility of the SNBTS is to provide an adequate supply of safe blood and blood products to meet patient needs in the prevention, treatment and diagnosis of disease and injury. This includes:

(a) the organisation, collection and storage of donations of whole blood or plasma;

(b) laboratory testing of donations to prevent transmissible disease, to determine blood group status and, in some cases, to provide cross-matching blood for transfusion;

(c) preparation of blood components and processing of donations for direct therapeutic application of plasma fractionation;

(d) provision of certain laboratory diagnostic services related to ante-natal care and other specialist areas;

(e) production and supply of reagents especially for immunohaematology, clinical bio-chemistry controls and organ matching.

13. The transfusion services work on two basic principles: that human blood and plasma is obtained only from voluntary unpaid donors; and that the health service should be self-sufficient in blood and blood products. And by

the adoption of component therapy (ie giving patients only the blood components they require therapeutically) the advantages of more effective and safer treatment are combined with the optimum use of blood.

14. The supply of blood and blood products depends upon the willingness of the public to donate blood (or plasma for certain products) and the resources devoted to collection and processing. The quantity of blood collected has increased steadily and was 54.9 donations per 1,000 population in 1978/79.

15. The demand for blood and blood products is determined by the range and quality of products available and by current clinical practice. A Working Group, appointed by DHSS in association with SHHD to study trends in demand into the mid-1980s, has concluded that a blood transfusion service which collected enough blood to provide the required amount of albumin and Factor VIII would have the primary material for the required quantities of other major blood components. Its calculations indicated that 50–60 annual donations per 1,000 population and a transfusion rate of 60 per cent red cell concentrates would provide the 200 gm of albumin per 1,000 population likely to be required each year. The current donation rate (see paragraph 14 above) is therefore within the recommended range, *but an increase towards the top of the range (ie of about 10 per cent) is desirable. The efficiency and effectiveness of processing of blood donations to meet the recognised targets for blood products should also be increased.*

16. The PFC was designed for the modern fractionation process, which is most effective and economical in long production runs. Shift working would therefore be necessary to produce the full benefits, but the current NHS terms and conditions of service have provided a constraint on achieving this.

17. *Anaesthetic services* primarily provide support for surgical and obstetric services, but consultant anaesthetists now have direct responsibility for patients in certain intensive therapy units and for clinics for those suffering from intractable pain.

18. There is no direct measure of the demand for or workload of the anaesthetic services. The number of surgical operations has been fairly steady over the 10 years to 1977, but a simple count cannot take fully into account the larger workload from the increasing complexity of many surgical procedures and the longer operating time for highly specialised operations now becoming more commonplace. The present procedures relating to the giving of dental anaesthesia have been giving rise to some anxiety. An NMCC/NDCC joint working party has been studying the problem and has recommended as

an ultimate objective that general anaesthesia, wherever required by a general dental practitioner, should be administered by specialist anaesthetic staff.

19. The numbers of anaesthetic staff have grown by over 16 per cent since NHS reorganisation with the number of consultants growing by 13 per cent, but this expansion appears to have done no more than keep pace with the increasing demand; and there appear to be problems of distribution between health boards. With a view to improving the distribution of staff, *consideration might be given to the question of financial incentives as a means of attracting anaesthetists to areas where recruitment is difficult.*

20. There are five *medical physics and bio-engineering* departments in Scotland, providing services routinely for health boards. In addition, certain specialised services are provided by the Department of Bio-engineering, Strathclyde University, by the Bio-engineering Unit, University of Edinburgh, at the Princess Margaret Rose Orthopaedic Hospital, Edinburgh, and by the Dundee Limb Fitting Centre.

21. These services provided by the five departments include scientific and technical advice and assistance to other health care professions where techniques used involve technology based on applied physics, electronic engineering, mechanical engineering, radiation physics, applied mathematics and computer science. In addition medical physics departments have routine clinical commitments in fields such as nuclear medicine, the servicing of electro-medical and scientific equipment, radiotherapy and ultrasonography. In some cases some staff may be permanently attached to clinical or laboratory units.

22. No statistics are collected centrally which would readily indicate the demand upon medical physics departments, but the increasing sophistication and proliferation of electro-medical and scientific equipment must increase their workload, as may the recent decision that these departments could properly assume responsibility for servicing and maintenance of such equipment in collaboration with hospital engineering departments. The increasing demand/workload is perhaps reflected in the increase in staff numbers. By September 1977 there were 116 physicists, a ratio of 22 per 1 million population, and 259 (whole-time equivalent) medical physics technicians.

23. There seem likely to be scientific developments in health care which will affect the work of medical physics departments. Whether these developments necessarily indicate a need for increased resources will be for consideration, especially as the number of physicists employed in Scotland seems to be

proportionately much higher than elsewhere in the UK (though this may at least in part be accounted for by the extent to which medical physicists in Scotland are staffing university medical schools). *As far as possible, changes and increases should be met from within existing resources.*

(ii) Ambulance service

24. The Scottish Ambulance Service (SAS) is a Division of the Common Services Agency (CSA), with its headquarters in Glasgow and eight ambulance areas covering the whole of Scotland, each in charge of a Chief Ambulance Officer and with a local ambulance committee. Its duty is to provide transport by ambulance or other means for 'persons suffering from illness or expectant or nursing mothers or other persons for whom such transport is reasonably required in order to avail themselves of any service under the NHS'. Except in an emergency, transport must be ordered by or on behalf of a doctor.

25. Of the patients for whom the SAS arranges transport, most go by road ambulance; some go by the Hospital Car Service (manned by volunteer drivers) or by a car hired by the SAS; a relatively small number are carried by the air ambulance service and a few by Ministry of Defence helicopters. Patients may also be provided by SAS expense with a seat on a scheduled air service in appropriate circumstances.

26. The number of patients carried by road vehicles in a normal year (ie one not disrupted by industrial action, etc) seems likely to be over 2 million, of whom rather more than one in three would be a stretcher case. The major part of the workload is patients using out-patient services and day hospitals and can therefore be planned in advance. Day hospitals impose a special burden in that ambulances are expected to be allocated specifically to the task and not to be diverted to emergency work. Difficulties in the development of day hospitals (as advocated in 'The Way Ahead') are being encountered through lack of the necessary transport, and we are attracted to the idea in the Programme Planning Group Report on Services for the Elderly that some other arrangement might be considered. One possibility is that the day hospital would provide its own transport.

27. The demand on the SAS seems certain to continue to increase but, as the greatest proportion of the increase will probably be in planned work (ie other than accident and emergency), the increase in resources can probably be proportionately less. Nevertheless, significant increases in financial resources

would seem to be necessary if the SAS is to meet the increasing demands in the same way as at present, and the pressure to recruit more ambulancemen to enable reductions in stand-by duty following a normal tour of day duty and to make greater use of double-manned ambulances (ie with both driver and attendant). *The decision by the Management Committee of the CSA that a review of the SAS be undertaken is to be welcomed, especially if the review is extensive enough to cover the question of arrangements for day hospital transport discussed in the preceding paragraph.*

Appendix 3

Preface to the Report of the Working Party on Health Priorities

We were appointed by the Planning Council in June 1975 'to review health priorities in Scotland and to recommend any changes required to make the most effective use of resources'. The Planning Council, at its meeting on 8 March 1978 agreed to a proposal by the Scottish Home and Health Department that we be asked to produce draft national guidelines for the Scottish Health Service for the 80s with emphasis on the period 1980–86, to replace those contained in the memorandum, 'The Health Service in Scotland: The Way Ahead', issued by the Secretary of State for Scotland in April 1976. The purpose of the latter was 'to describe the implications of the present economic situation for the National Health Service in Scotland, and to advise on priorities in the period 1976–80'.

In setting about this important task we have been conscious that it has to be tackled in a relatively broad way since, in general, national guidelines must be subject to local interpretation.

The main source of information on which we have based our proposals is the review of the Scottish Health Service prepared by the Scottish Home and Health Department's Health Service Planning Unit, which we have found to be a most useful document. In preparing the review, the Planning Unit took into account the several reports by the Programme Planning Groups set up by the Planning Council; we ourselves had the opportunity of studying all these reports, and we had oral presentations on many of them. The Programme Planning Groups were properly concerned only with their respective programmes and recommended what they considered should be done with these programmes. Our task was set in the wider context of the whole Health Service, and we therefore had to weigh in broad terms the competing claims on the resources likely to be available. We recognise that some of the Programme Planning Groups' recommendations, while commendable as long-term goals, will not be attainable within the period under consideration, because of the current financial constraint in which the Health Service, along with other public services, finds itself and because of the substantial additional resource implications, including professional staff, for which provision can only be made on a long timescale. We consider however that these recommendations, with their resource implications, provide strong arguments for allocation of additional funds to the Scottish Health Service when the financial climate improves.

Being aware that the Programme Planning Groups necessarily covered only part of the Scottish Health Service, we had earlier asked that the advisory bodies, in particular the National Medical and National Nursing and Mid-wifery Consultative Committees, be invited to assist us by considering priorities within the acute and maternity hospital services with a view to determining where expenditure should be maintained, increased or decreased, in the context of little or no growth. We derived great assistance from the reports we received from these two committees and the National Pharma-ceutical Consultative Committee, and from subsequent discussions with representatives of these committees.

We also considered that it would be helpful to have information on what health boards had in fact spent on particular health care programmes, as an indication of how far there had been a shift in emphasis towards those programmes accorded priority in 'The Way Ahead'. We therefore asked the Department to invite health boards to let us have analyses for the four financial years, 1974/75 to 1977/78. Most health boards had responded by the time we wrote this report, and although the time-scale was too short for us to evaluate fully the effect of 'The Way Ahead', the information from their returns provided us with a useful indication of what had happened over more than 90 per cent of the country since NHS reorganisation.

We have also studied the report of the Royal Commission on the National Health Service which was published in July 1979.

In accordance with our terms of reference we are, of course, concerned solely with priorities within the Scottish Health Service, but we are very much aware that there are many factors outside the Health Service which have a sub-stantial influence on the health status of the people of Scotland–housing standards, unemployment levels, etc. In addition, the load falling upon the Scottish Health Service will be increased to the extent that patients have to be admitted to or retained in hospital solely because suitable accommodation or supporting services outwith the Health Service are not available. These factors have necessarily influenced us in our deliberations.

We have had particular regard to the financial resources likely to be available for the Scottish Health Service, as indicated in the Public Expenditure

Surveys, and to estimates of the capital and net revenue costs that would be incurred in implementing the various recommendations in reports by Programme Planning Groups and National Consultative Committees and in meeting the objectives we ourselves have suggested for various programmes of health care.

The report is composed of seven chapters which fall naturally into two groups. The first three chapters are based on the information which was put to us, and they set out the recommendations we arrived at on the basis of this information. They are entitled:

    I.   The Need for Health Care
   II.   The Provision of Health Care
 III.   Provision of Resources: Manpower and Finance

The last four chapters bring together the recommendations in the earlier chapters, and deal with:

  IV.   Multiple Deprivation
   V.   Prevention
  VI.   Priorities
 VII.   Programme Objectives

In Chapters II and III of the draft report we have included various recommendations for evaluations of existing services or proposed new developments. We hope these can be carried out before the next planning round.

We have been forced to the conclusion that more suitable information is required for effective health service planning, in particular:

a.   Generally, more information needs to be sought on planning techniques and ways of determining priorities in health care;

b.   Better information on the health care needs of the population;

c.   Information on the stock of NHS building and facilities which would give an estimate of the amount of investment required to replace or upgrade those which are too dilapidated, or too obsolete in design, to meet generally accepted standards of provision ie in business parlance to allow for depreciation. At present some information is available on the age of hospitals but this does not take account of improvements and upgradings since the hospital was built;

d.   Better cost information related to activity data, in a form which would be used to assess the costs of proposed new developments in future plans;

e.   Similar information, probably in the form of programme budgets, which could be used to monitor progress towards meeting the national guidelines.

We are indebted to all those who have given us the benefit of their knowledge and experience. In particular, our thanks go to our secretary, Mr W. R. Miller, and to Mr J. Leithead and Mr A. W. Wallace.

J. G. Wallace
Chairman
Working Party on Health Priorities
May 1980

Membership of Working Party on Health Priorities

CHAIRMAN

| Mr J. G. Wallace | *formerly Member, Lothian Health Board* |

MEMBERS

Professor Sir John Crofton	*Emeritus Professor of Respiratory Diseases and Tuberculosis, University of Edinburgh (appointed 1 September 1976)*
Dr G. D. Forwell	*Chief Administrative Medical Officer, Greater Glasgow Health Board*
Dr J. H. Grant	*Director, Health Service Planning Unit, Scottish Home and Health Department (appointed 3 July 1978)*
Dr M. A. Heasman	*Director, Information Services Division, Common Services Agency*
Mr J. B. Hume	*Under Secretary, Scottish Home and Health Department (appointed 12 July 1977)*
Mr W. P. Lawrie	*Assistant Secretary, Scottish Home and Health Department*
Dr I. S. MacDonald	*Deputy Chief Medical Officer, Scottish Home and Health Department*
Professor J. D. McEwen	*Professor of Dentistry, University of Dundee*
Miss D. A. McLauchlan	*Chief Area Nursing Officer, Ayrshire and Arran Health Board*
Miss E. K. McNaught	*Deputy Chief Nursing Officer, Scottish Home and Health Department*
Mr J. A. M. Mitchell	*Under Secretary, Scottish Home and Health Department (resigned 31 October 1976)*
Mr R. Mitchell	*Secretary, Fife Health Board*

Mr G. H. Mooney	*Director, Health Economics Research Unit, University of Aberdeen (appointed 29 July 1977)*
Dr D. M. Pendreigh	*formerly Director, Health Service Planning Unit, Scottish Home and Health Department; now Senior Lecturer, Department of Community Medicine, University of Edinburgh*
Mr A. L. Rennie	*Under Secretary, Scottish Home and Health Department (appointed 1 November 1976, resigned 30 June 1977)*
Mr L. M. Williams	*Treasurer, Lothian Health Board*

ASSESSORS

Dr M. Ashley-Miller	*Director, Chief Scientist Office, Scottish Home and Health Department*
Mr T. D. Hunter	*Secretary, Scottish Health Service Planning Council*
Mr J. Leithead	*Senior Principal, Health Service Planning Unit, Scottish Home and Health Department (until May 1977)*
Mr A. W. Wallace	*Principal, Health Service Planning Unit, Scottish Home and Health Department (from July 1978)*

SECRETARY

| Mr R. Mowat | *Principal, Secretariat, Scottish Health Service Planning Council (until July 1977)* |
| Mr W. R. Miller | *Principal, Health Service Planning Unit, Scottish Home and Health Department (from December 1977)* |

Printed in Scotland by Her Majesty's Stationery Office at HMSO Press, Edinburgh
Dd 0630400/4068 K44 12/80 (17507)